Evidence-based Management
A practical guide for health professionals

Rosemary Stewart
Templeton College
University of Oxford

Radcliffe Medical Press

Radcliffe Medical Press Ltd
18 Marcham Road
Abingdon
Oxon OX14 1AA
United Kingdom

www.radcliffe-oxford.com
The Radcliffe Medical Press electronic catalogue and online ordering facility.
Direct sales to anywhere in the world.

British Library Cataloguing in Publication Data

A catalogue record for this book is available from the British Library.

ISBN 1 85775 458 1

Typeset by Acorn Bookwork, Salisbury, Wiltshire
Printed and bound by TJ International Ltd, Padstow, Cornwall

Contents

About the author   iv
Acknowledgements   v
List of figures   vi

Introduction   1

1   An overview of evidence-based management   5

2   Managing the job   29

3   Using information and knowledge   43

4   Are we doing a good job?   73

5   Improving decision making   93

6   Learning to practise evidence-based management   119

7   Organisational culture   143

8   In conclusion   157

Index   159

About the author

Rosemary Stewart's career has been in management research and teaching, combined for seven years with managing. Her doctorate was at the London School of Economics and she has an Hon DPhil from Uppsala University, Sweden.

She was a Fellow in Organisational Behaviour at Templeton College, University of Oxford, and is now an Honorary Fellow and Co-director of the Oxford Health Care Management Institute at Templeton College. Her research has covered a wide range of subjects and organisations in industry, commerce, local government and the NHS. Her main research interests are in managerial work and behaviour and management in the NHS. She has run workshops for many years for NHS chief executives and, currently, for chairs. She has lectured in many parts of the world.

She has written more than a dozen books. Her best known is *The Reality of Management* (Butterworth-Heinemann, 1999), now in its third edition, and its companion *The Reality of Organizations*. A specifically NHS book is *Leading in the NHS: a practical guide* (Macmillan, 1995).

Acknowledgements

I am indebted to all those who provided the material for the case studies. I am particularly grateful for their willingness to answer points of clarification, even though they were very busy, and to check what I wrote.

The book has been much improved by the penetrating criticisms and very helpful suggestions made by a friend, Trevor Owen CBE. He drew on his experience in senior posts in industry and as the former chairman of a leading NHS trust to do so, and on his own skill as the author of a perceptive and very readable management book. My husband, Professor Ioan James, took time from writing a book on Remarkable Physicists to scan this alien material and to make helpful criticisms. Of course, the responsibility for the views expressed and the remaining defects is mine.

List of figures

Figure 1.1 Aids and obstacles to practising evidence-based management.

Figure 2.1 Model of a managerial job.

Figure 3.1 Requirements of good information.

Figure 3.2 Obstacles to obtaining and using information.

Figure 7.1 Is the culture favourable to evidence-based management?

Introduction

This book is aimed to be of practical help to managers – the word 'manager' is used to include all those with responsibility for other people, whatever their professional background. In a time of rapid change, managers are less able to rely on previous knowledge and experience; instead they may have to look for the best available evidence to help in decision making.

Evidence-based means that your decisions should, as far as possible, be based on evidence. The idea that this matters comes from evidence-based medicine. It is easy to see why evidence-based medicine is increasingly accepted as the right way to practise medicine. As patients, we want our doctors to use the best evidence on the treatment of particular diseases. But are the same ideas relevant to management? I found this question intriguing. I wrote an article about evidence-based management for the *Health Service Journal* in 1998 and went on thinking about the answer to the question. My conclusion is that the ideas are useful for managers because it is a desirable way of thinking, but that it is more difficult to practise evidence-based management than evidence-based medicine.

This book aims to make it easier to practise evidence-based management. It is designed for two different kinds of readers: those who want a quick practical guide to how to practise evidence-based management and those who are willing to give more time to understanding it. The first kind of reader should look at the tables and figures and their explanations, the summaries of each chapter and the points on how to apply evidence-based management at the end of Chapters 3–7. Most managers should also find it helpful to read Chapter 2. To avoid the challenge: 'What is your evidence?', I have cited more references than I usually would in a book for managers.

The ideas behind evidence-based management are relevant to managers in most organisations, but they are particularly relevant to an organisation as large and complex as the National Health Service, where intuition and entrepreneurial instinct have much less scope than in a small trading company. There are two other reasons why the NHS is a suitable focus for this book: one, any manager who works in the health services will know about the growing emphasis on evidence-based medicine and so the idea of evidence-based management will be more acceptable; two, the NHS is, relative to many large companies, rather weak in its concern for evidence and in its monitoring of operations. However, readers from other organisations, particularly in the public sector, will also find that the book can be helpful to them, particularly the 'How to improve' sections at the end of each chapter.

Chapter 1 defines evidence-based management and contrasts it with evidence-based medicine. Since the growth of evidence-based medicine is one of the reasons for an interest in evidence-based management, it is useful to explore the similarities and differences between the two. It is easier to practise evidence-based medicine, but there are still problems in doing so that provide useful lessons for the practice of evidence-based management. One is that evidence is less concrete than its protagonists claim, another is that what is accepted as evidence depends on the attitudes of the people involved.

Many different factors affect the practice of evidence-based management; some make it easier and some make it harder. These are illustrated in a diagram. Much of the book is about how to reduce the obstacles to its practice.

Chapter 2 starts with the prior requirement for the practice of evidence-based management, managing your job well. Unless you can do that, you will be too harassed and distracted to be able to consider, far less practise, evidence-based management. The chapter draws on the studies of managerial work and behaviour to show what you can do to manage your job better.

Chapter 3 is about getting the information you need for making decisions, and for alerting you to problems needing attention. It explains why knowledge management has developed as a new subject and what it contributes. Chapter 4 is about the need for good monitoring, since this is an essential aspect of evidence-based management, and how to improve it.

Chapter 5 describes the nature of decision making and what research has shown about the obstacles to making effective decisions, which includes their successful implementation. It also discusses what research can tell us about how to improve decision making. Chapter 6 is about what you need to learn to practise evidence-based management. Many suggestions are made for how to improve this learning.

Chapter 7 discusses how organisational culture influences whether managers in an organisation are interested in practising evidence-based management. It shows how to assess this aspect of the culture of the organisation and what are the characteristics of an organisational culture that is supportive of evidence-based management. It describes the criticisms of the culture of the NHS.

Many examples are provided to illustrate various ways in

which an evidence-based management approach can be applied. These case studies have two purposes: first, to illustrate what is being said by giving a specific example; second, to encourage readers to think critically about their own practice and whether they have anything to learn from the case study. All but one of the examples are drawn from the health service, but the lessons from them are usually also applicable to other organisations. As patients or potential patients, we have an additional reason for being interested in health management case studies.

1

An overview of evidence-based management

Evidence-based management is primarily an attitude of mind.

What is evidence-based management? Why should managers practise it? These are the questions that a first chapter should answer. It will also look at what can be learnt from the development of evidence-based medicine, and at what can be done to overcome the obstacles to practising evidence-based management.

Managers would benefit from practising evidence-based management because:

- it is a way of overcoming some common management failings
- the rapid changes affecting organisations reduce the value of experience as a guide to managing
- there is a revolution in the importance and accessibility of information

- the development of evidence-based medicine has shown the way.

What is evidence-based management?

There are two answers to this question. For the first, the widely used definition of evidence-based medicine:

The conscientious, explicit and judicious use of current best evidence in making decisions about the care of individual patients.[1]

can be modified to:

The conscientious, explicit and judicious use of current best evidence in making decisions.

The words 'conscientious', 'explicit' and 'judicious' in the definition are each important for good practice. 'Conscientious' means that managers will consider what evidence is relevant for a decision and, where necessary, will search for it. 'Explicit' means that the nature of the evidence on which a decision is to be based will be examined and not taken for granted. 'Judicious' means a careful examination of the nature and reliability of the evidence.

Many decisions will be routine ones that are taken on the basis of experience without any search for more information. Evidence-based management is relevant to the more important and unusual decisions, but as in medicine, you should check periodically to see that your habitual experience-based decisions are still relevant.

The first answer to the question: 'What is evidence-based management?' is too narrow and too academic to be of much help to the manager. A broader answer is also needed. This is given at the head of the chapter: 'Evidence-based management is primarily an attitude of mind'. This shows itself by a questioning approach, which asks the following questions.

- How should we assess performance?
- What questions should we be asking ourselves about our performance? 'Our' may be a team, or any organisational unit, large or small.
- What kind of information do we need to answer each question?
- Where and how can we find it?
- What is the most reliable way of getting it?
- What can we realistically do to improve our performance?
- How should we monitor our performance?
- Is the information that we are using good evidence? What may make it inaccurate?
- Is it important to try and improve the quality of the evidence? Have we the time and resources to do so? If not, what allowances should we make for possible inaccuracies?

Many aspects of evidence-based management are part of good management, and are called planning, organising, monitoring and implementing, but they may be neglected, or poorly done. An emphasis on evidence-based management can be used to give a new focus to tackle these common management failings – failings that now matter more because experience is less often a good guide than in the past.

The idea of evidence-based management can be applied in any organisation, but it is easier to do so in the public sector because information can be shared more freely than in the private sector. This difference is illustrated in a US article about evidence-based management in healthcare[2] which argues the need for evidence-based management cooperatives to overcome the reluctance to share information.

Lessons from evidence-based medicine?

Many readers from the health services will be familiar with the term 'evidence-based medicine', and even know the common abbreviation EBM – pity it has been appropriated and so cannot be used for evidence-based management! Managers from other sectors may not. The simplest explanation of evidence-based medicine is that it is a way of helping, and persuading, clinicians to use the most up-to-date evidence on the best way to treat a particular disease. To be used, clinicians must know about it, so a variety of ways of telling them have been developed. There is the Cochrane Centre, which provides up-to-date summaries of the latest evidence; there is a journal, *Evidence-based Medicine*. Guidelines or protocols are also produced by different medical groups, usually after considerable discussion and consultation, particularly for common diseases where there is wide agreement about what is the best evidence. These may give very detailed prescriptions for how to treat a particular disease.

A lot of effort has been spent in the UK and the US, and other countries, from the 1990s onwards to encourage the practice of evidence-based medicine. As a 2001 doctoral thesis comparing US/UK initiatives in this area says:

> *Evidence-Based Medicine (EBM) has for the past several years been viewed by many politicians, managers and clinicians as the magic key to changing clinical practice in the US and UK.*[3]

The enthusiasm from policy makers arose not just from the desire that doctors should practise evidence-based medicine, but also in the expectation, especially in the US, that doing so could make for economies to help offset the alarming rise in the costs of using new medical discoveries.

There has been a lot of enthusiastic support for the idea of EBM, but also considerable controversy. This has focused on the relative importance of evidence and experience, on what is meant by 'evidence'[4] and, particularly in the US, on a concern that it was finance driven. Specific concerns are:

- how generally applicable is the research? Is it relevant to different kinds of patients and to different situations?
- the relative importance of research results compared with experience in deciding on what treatment is appropriate for a particular patient
- that evidence-based medicine can encourage a false sense of scientific accuracy and objectivity, when medicine is still an art where experience is important
- that protocols based on the research may be used too rigidly to allocate resources and used by nurses in circumstances where more medical experience is required to assess whether the protocol is appropriate for the particular patient.

Researchers who did four in-depth case studies of clinical changes in one region of the NHS concluded that medical evidence is much less clear-cut than discussions of evidence-based medicine often suggest:

> *Our research suggests that scientific evidence is not a clear, accepted and bounded source. There is no such entity as 'the body of evidence'.... Much of what is called evidence is, in fact, a contested domain, constituted in the debates and controversies of opposing viewpoints in search of ever more compelling arguments.*[5]

The researchers emphasise that evidence does not speak for itself, but must always be seen in context, which includes the local ideas, practices and attitudes of professionals. **Both in management and in medicine there is a need to be precise in talking about the evidence being considered: what specifically is it evidence of?**

The main lesson that those who want to practise evidence-based management should learn from the experience of evidence-based medicine is that evidence is socially determined, that is, it can only be used as evidence if other people accept it as such. A powerful top manager in a large technical company used to say when he disagreed with arguments being put forward: 'My facts are better than yours'. Another lesson is that one should not have too optimistic a view about the nature of evidence, thinking of it as hard facts, but rather as the best that we can find for our purposes.

Comparing evidence-based medicine and evidence-based management

There are major differences between the problems faced by clinicians and managers, but the similarities make some of the lessons from evidence-based medicine relevant to evidence-based management.

Similarities in the practice of evidence-based medicine and the practice of evidence-based management

- The need for evidence-based practice has become much greater for both clinicians and managers because of the rapidity of change affecting their work. It has also become greater because doctors and managers in the public sector, particularly chief executives, are held more accountable for their actions than in the past.
- New developments in medicine and in management, and changes in the political, social, economic and technical environment, mean learning about their implications.

- Clinicians and managers face a similar difficulty in the time pressure to take decisions; both have to decide when a decision requires more thought and the collection of more evidence.
- Both medicine and management are an art, where intuition and skill are important, as well as a science. Despite the widespread growth in MBAs, management remains more of an art than a science in that it is still possible to practise it, and to practise it successfully, without formal management qualifications. However, an increasing number of managers and would-be managers see an MBA degree as a necessary step for advancement. To have one helps in understanding the nature of managerial problems, the available techniques and the environment within which the manager works.

There are common factors that make evidence-based practice easier:

- good time management so that clinicians and managers are able to consider whether more evidence is necessary, rather than being forced by time pressures to rely too much on their experience when making decisions. Both clinicians and managers should do their job in a thoughtful way, which is much harder to do if they fail to manage their time
- a willingness to reflect on your practice
- an interest in evidence and in keeping up to date, although the latter is more important for clinicians
- easy availability of relevant evidence, which is also more important for clinicians
- working with people who value learning to improve and are willing to examine current practice critically, that is, working in a culture that is supportive of evidence-based practice.

Differences in the practice of evidence-based medicine and the practice of evidence-based management

- *The rationale for evidence-based practice.* Evidence-based medicine starts from a concern that individual clinicians should be using the most up-to-date medical knowledge in their practice, and the fear that the rapid development of medical knowledge and technologies has made it much harder to do so. For managers, the problem is different as the body of knowledge is not developing nearly as rapidly. Their problem is keeping up to date with the speed of change affecting organisations and understanding what information is relevant to a particular decision. It is also learning to think critically about their work and that of their organisation.
- *The nature of the problems being addressed.* Managerial problems are murkier, less structured, less familiar than many, but not all, medical problems, therefore understanding the nature of the problem is often harder.
- *The nature of the evidence.* Medical evidence is quantitative, based on the results of research following the agreed ways of testing the effects of a new treatment. In management, it is harder than in medicine to assess what evidence is necessary and how to find it, and it is often more difficult to know how to interpret it. Also there is no equivalently rigorous research information to inform decision making.
- *The methods available to facilitate evidence-based practice.* Readily and quickly available summaries of the latest evidence on diagnosis and treatment and the development of clinical guidelines and protocols, which describe the appropriate treatment for a particular disease, are practical methods for making evidence-based medicine easier to practise. There can, for the reasons given above, be no

equivalent in management. Ways of encouraging the practice of evidence-based management have to be much more diverse.

- *The value attached to experience.* Experience counts for more in medicine than in management because the problems are more repetitive.
- *Who makes the decision.* Doctors will usually be making decisions individually, whereas managerial decisions are often taken collectively.
- *The types of decision made at different levels of seniority.* There is much more difference in management than in medicine between the kinds, and the time span, of decisions made at different levels.
- *The timescale of decision making.* In medicine, decisions about diagnosis and treatment will usually be made quickly; in management, there is often much more scope for prolonging decision making to try and arrive at the best decision. The fact that management decisions are often made by a group also contributes to a lengthy process of decision making.

What is evidence in management?

This book takes a broad view of what is evidence in management, like that given in an article on evidence-based management:

> *'Evidence' is defined as empirical data that is logically ordered and relates to specified assumptions.*[6]

The final part of the definition, 'specified assumptions', is particularly important because the need to spell out what they are can easily be overlooked. In Chapter 6, we shall come back to the need to understand the assumptions being made.

The 'current best evidence' (from the definition given earlier) for management can be very diverse. It can be hard quantitative data, like expenditure over the last year, the sales figures for a particular product in France during the last quarter, or the pattern of hospital admissions over the last year. It can be data that are still quantitative but more subject to error, like the projected costs of a new building, which often prove to be unreliable. Then there are data where the utility is very dependent on the assumptions made about them. This is true of much information about people and their reactions. An example is the conclusions that can be drawn from an interview survey of employees' reactions to a proposed change: is it, for example, correct to assume that the employees told the interviewer what they really thought? That what they said at the time of the interview is still their opinion?

The broad view of evidence in evidence-based management contrasts with a narrow view like that taken by Axelsson, a Swedish professor, who sees it as encouraging and making use of research into good management practice:

Evidence-based management means that health care managers should learn to search for and critically appraise evidence from management research as a basis for their practice.[7]

The opportunities for the practice of evidence-based management would indeed be rare if this narrow view was adopted! Management decisions may have to be taken quickly. Even when there is time, there is not much research into good management practice, except that which provides broad guidance in organisational behaviour. I say this reluctantly as I have been doing research into management practice all my working life! Alastair Hewison, in an article in the *Journal of Nursing Management*, 'Evidence-based medicine: what about evidence-based management?', ends with a plea for more research into management in action and the principles under-lying it to provide the knowledge base for effective management.[8] More management research, particularly into the causes of particular problems and the effects of policies, should be encouraged, but even if it is, the opportunities for management decision making to be based on research will remain much more limited than in medicine. The attempt to find underlying principles was abandoned with the discovery of how organisations varied and the discrediting of the classical school of management, which had produced principles of good management.

A core idea of evidence-based management is that managers, and clinicians in their managerial role, will seek to base their decisions on the best evidence available. The scientific standards required for evidence-based medicine are rarely feasible in management, or even necessary. What is needed is information that is useful in reaching management decisions and as reliable as possible within the constraints of the situation.

What is good evidence?

In evidence-based medicine there is a gold standard for determining what is good evidence, the randomised controlled trial (RCT) or even perhaps now the review of RCTs. The standard for managers who want to practise evidence-based management is less clear and has to be more pragmatic. Which disciplines might be helpful? Evidence is discussed by philosophers, lawyers and psychologists. In philosophy, there are different schools of thought about what we can know, but they are unlikely to be useful to the manager. Lawyers are more helpful, although they have a special interest in what should count as evidence in court.

Whether information is sufficiently reliable to be treated as evidence is a subject that is central to those writing about the law of evidence. It is not a central concern for managers, but it is still worth thinking about what kinds of information one is dealing with and how reliable they are. One danger is accepting as evidence information that is inaccurate or false: figures that have been massaged – a politer term than falsified – to give a better impression than the reality; research that has failed to explore relevant aspects and explanations that are taken as factual without checking. Another danger is not looking for corroborative evidence. Here it can be helpful to remember the different types of evidence that might be explored. These include: research, recorded experience of others, lessons from the organisation's past and asking how other people have tackled a similar problem.

Psychology is the most useful discipline for managers because psychologists and social psychologists have researched how people think individually and in groups, including how individuals can behave differently in groups from how they would on their own and express different views from their private ones. Other findings from psychological and social psychological research that can be useful to managers are discussed later.

A useful warning that comes from much social research is that it is easy to believe something that is not true, to accept an explanation of a problem that is incorrect or to have very selective memories. I remember examples in my own research. Two case studies, one of the introduction of a successful new product and the other of a failure, came from the same well-known company. They were written up anonymously, that is, all the details were there but the name was changed. I gave the two case studies to the managing director. He recognised and cleared the successful one but said of the failure: 'Why have you shown this to me'? He had not recognised it! Another example was of the explanation that managers gave for the failure of a new product: that they had chosen a bad time of month to launch it because sales were always low then, even though their records showed that this was not true.

Evidence-based medicine as a link to evidence-based management

Two interesting examples are given below of how experience in encouraging evidence-based medicine has led to applying the same evidence-based thinking to management issues. Both examples illustrate a way of thinking that can, and should, be applied more generally in management.

The first example comes from the Birmingham Specialist Community Health NHS Trust, which was formed by a merger of two trusts. The merger was seen as providing an ideal opportunity for assessment and review. The new trust aims to develop a critical approach to decision making and a systematic approach to issues by:

- conducting baseline assessments to find out what is happening and how it is happening
- agreeing what should be happening, based on evidence wherever this is available
- drawing up action plans, identifying what has to be done, by whom and the timescale.

The trust has produced a knowledge management strategy to support the development of critical appraisal skills. The importance attached to these skills is shown by the fact that the professional staff in the clinical governance department, formerly the clinical audit department, have undertaken MScs in related subjects, such as health information science, evidence-based practice and quality, and all have a certificate in project management. All staff, including consultants, have appraisals that centre round setting measurable objectives.

The projects carried out in 1999–2001 in the new trust, and earlier in South Birmingham Community NHS Trust, one of the merged trusts, illustrate the practice of evidence-based management applied to ways of improving the quality of care. All projects followed the three-point plan given above, and included field research. One project was the development of key performance indicators for the seven clinical director-ates of the new trust, identifying where improvements are needed. Another was an audit of medical record keeping, which is described in Chapter 4, pp. 83–4. There were several projects on identifying the needs of particular ethnic groups, one on Asian first-time parents and another on Yemeni elders, which is briefly described in Chapter 4, p. 76. Another project was on ward-based falls prevention.

The second example comes from the Berkshire Health Authority, which took the unusual step of reviewing the evidence base of the commissioning decisions (those about what forms of treatment are to be financed). It found that only a third of them were based on evidence of effectiveness from RCTs and systematic reviews, which are the basis for evidence-based medicine. One of the actions taken from the findings of this study was to set up a method of taking diffi-cult decisions about priorities for treatment in a robust and evidence-based way. Details of the study and the resulting action are given at the end of this chapter.

These are two examples of organisations where evidence-based management is taken seriously. Both can be helpful as exemplars, but we also need to understand what factors make it easier to practise evidence-based management and what makes it difficult to do so.

Influences on evidence-based management

Practising evidence-based management can be difficult. It is easier to do so well if one understands what helps and what hinders its practice. These are the personal factors, the nature of the job and the organisational context. The relevant characteristics of each are listed in Box 1.1.

Box 1.1:   Influences on the practice of evidence-based management

Personal	*Job*	*Context*
Ways of thinking	Workload	Organisational culture
Approach to the job	Time pressures	Rapidity of change
Education	Kinds of decisions	Political and
Experience	Information:	competitive
	— volume	
	— availability	
	— quality	
	— boss(es)' expectations	

In Box 1.1, under the heading 'personal', are the personality characteristics and the education and experience that help to determine how interested managers are likely to be in evidence-based management and how easy or difficult they will find it to appraise evidence critically. How the individual sees and judges what is happening is an aspect of personality – readers who have taken the Myers Briggs test will be familiar with the idea that people interpret the world differently and will know their own strengths and weaknesses in how they do so. How managers think about their job will also influence how they tackle it.

Some managers are more thoughtful and analytical than others and will find the idea of evidence-based management appealing. The very pragmatic manager will find it antipathetic. If you are like that, but are willing to accept that the idea of evidence-based management has merit, you should make use of those who are more naturally analytical to help in asking the searching questions that may be needed to clarify what you are talking about. Even if you are not analytically minded you can still make use of the simple questions: What? When? Where? How? and Who? You should also read the 'How to improve' section at the end of each chapter, as you are likely to find some suggestions that will appeal to you.

One of the most important obstacles to practising evidence-based management is an inability to manage the job, so that the manager is overwhelmed by work and has no time for reflection – the next chapter covers this. Another obstacle is a view of management as being mainly intuitive, because then there is no need to look for evidence. An undue belief in the value of your own judgement is also a handicap.

The kind of education that you have had can be an aid or an obstacle. An analytical education, particularly a training in critical thinking and in the evaluation of evidence, is an aid. Those who have had that will find that evidence-based management is a natural way of thinking and will only need suggestions for how to practise it better and information about how to do so. Little education or a very practical one may be an obstacle because you have not been trained to think analytically and evaluatively. Like many obstacles, a poor education, or one that was very practically oriented, can be counteracted. You can, for example, make use of your own ways of learning: you may be a person who can learn far more by a visit to see how other people are handling the same problem than by reading about it or listening to a lecture on it.

There are jobs where the pressures of work and the time pressures imposed by superiors make it very difficult to practise evidence-based management well – none where it is impossible because it is an attitude of mind that can be applied in all but emergency situations. The job may be a very hectic one. It can also be worryingly controversial, depending on powerful stakeholders' attitudes to, and expectations of, the jobholder. The types of decisions that have to be taken may include those where there is little evidence and even the best available is ambiguous. The jobholder may also be swamped by information and demands for action. In sum, there are jobs where it is very hard to practise evidence-based management, although even in those, good habits can be developed, such as asking simple questions: 'How do we know?', 'What is the evidence for that?' Or prompts, like 'Let's try and learn from that mistake before we forget.'

The organisational context can help or hinder the practice of evidence-based management. It will affect how easy it is for managers to get the information they need, including how willing other staff are to share information and to try to look objectively at problems. For the practice of evidence-based management, the key thing to remember about organisations is that they are systems composed of different parts that interact, so that the repercussions of a decision about one part of the organisation can have wider effects than had been anticipated. The organisational culture is likely to be the most important aspect of the organisational context for the practice of evidence-based management; it is discussed in Chapter 7.

How these different factors can help or hinder the practice of evidence-based management is shown in Figure 1.1. Subsequent chapters will draw on relevant research for lessons on how to overcome the difficulties. It helps to assess the extent to which the influences are aids or obstacles for you, so that you can decide what you can do to make good use of the aids and to reduce or counteract the obstacles.

An obstacle, which is a by-product of the lack of attention to evidence-based management, is the shortage of applied research into management, particularly into evaluating outcomes of decisions and different ways of tackling similar problems. This is hard to do for new policies in the public sector because the research results may be politically sensitive and evaluation may be unpopular, and even if it is carried

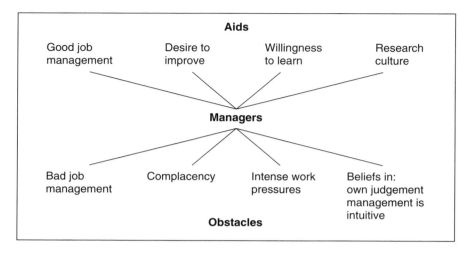

Figure 1.1   Aids and obstacles to practising evidence-based management.

out, may be suppressed if the results are critical of current policy. In the private sector, unwelcome results of research can more easily be made anonymous.

Research in the following areas helps us to understand what makes it easier and what makes it harder to practise evidence-based management and what can be done to strengthen the former and reduce the latter:

- managerial work and behaviour for an understanding of the nature of managerial jobs, how managers work in practice and the differences in managerial behaviour
- information management and the newer field of knowledge management, which is explained in Chapter 3
- decision making for studies of decision making in practice, including the role of internal politics
- psychology and social psychology for what it shows about how people think and behave
- organisational culture for how this affects behaviour, including what is judged to be important.

Lessons from these studies help to provide the evidence behind the following chapters.

What managers can achieve if they base their decisions on evidence as well as on traditional criteria is the difference between an organisation that works – just – and an organisation of which they can be proud. The subsequent chapters show how this can be done.

Summary

The practice of evidence-based management is increasingly necessary for managers to cope successfully in the rapidly changing world.

Two answers are given to the question: 'What is evidence-based management?' The first is to modify the most widely used definition of evidence-based medicine so that it becomes: 'The conscientious, explicit and judicious use of current best evidence in making decisions'. In management, a broad view must be taken of what is meant by current best evidence.

The second answer is that evidence-based management is primarily a questioning attitude of mind. Examples were given of the kinds of questions that an evidence-based manager would be asking in order to get the information needed and to assess its reliability. The same approach is also a part of good management, but one that is too often neglected. The practice of evidence-based management can provide the impetus to overcome this neglect.

Evidence-based medicine and evidence-based management were compared to see what lessons can be learnt from the experience of the former. The main warning from that experience is that evidence is often not as firm as its protagonists claim, and that what is accepted as evidence is affected by the views of the people concerned.

An understanding of the factors that help or hinder the

practice of evidence-based management, which are shown in Figure 1.1, can make it easier to practise it successfully.

Two examples were given of how experience in evidence-based medicine had been used as the basis for practising evidence-based management.

Details of linked Berkshire Health Authority cases

Reviewing evidence base for commissioning decisions

This case is included because:
- it brings together evidence-based medicine and evidence-based management
- it is unusual in being a study of the evidence base of past decisions
- these decisions were ones where better evidence was available than for many decisions
- yet only a third of the decisions were considered evidence based.

Objective To investigate the proportion of health policy and management commissioning decisions made in one district health authority (population 770 000) that were based on evidence of effectiveness from RCTs and systematic reviews. (Commissioning decisions are those about what forms of treatment are to be funded.)

Background The study was carried out in 1998 by members of the public health department because they wanted to understand how much use was being made of evidence in taking decisions by the authority, so that they could take this further.

Method A survey was made of three planning documents in 1997–98 from the district health authority and primary care purchasing pilots in Berkshire to identify planning statements. Effectiveness questions were constructed from these statements and used to search for evidence from systematic reviews and RCTs in the Cochrane Library (Issue 4, 1998), which is the centre for information for evidence-based medicine.

Findings One hundred and twenty four planning decisions were identified and nearly two thirds of these concerned how the health services were organised and delivered for patients. The study showed that 42 decisions (33.9%) were considered to be evidence based using the method described above; for a further 18 decisions (14.5%) evidence was identified which was equivocal or did not support the decision.

Subsequent actions:
- developed a training programme in critical appraisal skills for managers in the health authority to increase their ability to analyse and understand evidence from the literature
- the development described in the next case study.

Evaluation of a new prioritisation process

This case is included because:
- it is an evaluation of a new process for recommending priorities to the health authority board
- it is one of the actions resulting from the findings of the previous case study about the inadequate use of evidence in decisions
- a review was carried out among members of the Priorities Committee to check the extent to which they thought the new process met its five aims; recommendations based on this review were made to the Priorities Committee.

Background and objectives The Priorities Committee was set up in the latter part of 1999 to decide how to make difficult decisions about NHS funding of particular treatments in a robust and evidence-based way, with the following aims:
- representation of stakeholders across the country: purchasers, providers and users of healthcare
- transparency
- accountability

- due process (consistent application of the ethical framework)
- effects on resource utilisation.

The Priorities Committee produces policy statements for its approach to the funding of particular forms of treatment. Each describes the particular treatment and the information about the evidence base for its effectiveness. It then gives its recommendations for the priority, by applying its ethical framework to the evidence for a treatment, and for what conditions, and what further action the Committee should take.

The Committee produced 31 evidence-based policies, resulting in a saving of £90 000 in the first year, from reduced activity in 'low-priority treatments'. Twenty four members of the Committee were interviewed at the end of the first year about their views on the working of the Committee in relation to its five aims. These interviews showed some failings in communication and in understanding of the process among some members, as well as a failure to clearly share accountability between members. It also gave an approximate figure for the first year's opportunity cost. A number of recommendations were made to the Committee to improve its working, including establishing a system to monitor the implementation of policies across all NHS organisations in Berkshire.

Berkshire is now leading a region-wide priorities network so that the learning from the application of an ethical framework to evidence-based information can enable a health system to improve the cost-effectiveness of the local health services.

References

1 Sackett D, Rosenberg W, Gray J, Haynes R, Richardson W (1996) Evidence-based medicine: what it is and what it isn't. *BMJ.* **312**: 71–2.
2 Kovner AR, Elton JJ, Billings J, Short JH *et al.* (2000) Evidence-based management/commentaries/reply. *Front Health Serv Mgmt.* **16**(4): 3–46.
3 Chambers D (2001) An Exploration of the Influences on Evidence-Based Change to Clinical Practice: a com-

parative study of US/UK health care initiatives. DPhil thesis, University of Oxford, p. 3.

4   Evans R, Haines A (eds) (2000) *Implementing Evidence-based Changes in Healthcare*. Radcliffe Medical Press, Oxford. A good discussion of the lessons learnt from trying to apply research evidence in practice.

5   Wood M, Ferlie E, Fitzgerald L (1998) Achieving clinical behaviour change: a case of becoming indeterminate. *Soc Sci Med*. **47**: 1729–38.

6   Kovner *et al.* (2000) op. cit., p. 7.

7   Axelsson R (1998) Towards evidence-based health care management. *Int J Health Plan Mgmt*. **13**: 307–17.

8   Hewison A (1997) Evidence-based medicine: what about evidence-based management? *J Nurs Mgmt*. **5**(4): 196–7.

2

Managing the job

Steering or swept along?

You can only practise evidence-based management if you are managing the job: if you are constantly under pressure, rushing from one appointment to another and switching frenetically between problems you are not managing the job. The first step towards practising evidence-based management is to run the job rather than the job running you. Research into what managers do shows that in many managers' jobs it is difficult to resist being carried along by what is happening around you and by your appointments diary, which is likely to be filled with meetings. A few managers are very good at shaping the job and managing their time, some are very bad at doing so and most could improve. This chapter is about how to manage the job. Those managers who have nothing to learn about this – and there are managers of whom this is true – can skip this chapter.

There has been a lot of research, some of it by observation, into what managers are doing and how they are doing it. Obviously managers' jobs differ, but there are similarities in what managers are doing across a wide variety of jobs. The similarities that are relevant for this book are those that make it hard to practise evidence-based management. First is the fact that, apart from formal meetings, many activities are very short ones, lasting only a few minutes as the manager is switching between different problems and people. The fragmented nature of much managerial work was first identified by a Swedish professor, Sune Carlson, in the early 1950s, in a study of managing directors. Subsequent studies show that it remains a striking feature of managerial work.[1] Another common feature is the amount of time spent with other people: in most jobs at least two-thirds of time and in some operational management jobs as much as 90%. These two characteristics are related because it is people with queries, requests and problems who cause much of the fragmentation. They also contribute to the seductions of management that make it hard to be an effective and efficient manager.

Seductions of management

The buzz from busyness

Being busy can be pleasurable. For practical people, being busy can be particularly enjoyable, and managers tend to be practical people who prefer practice to theory: they like getting things done and sorting out problems. Most managers' jobs in organisations today are busy ones and it is all too easy to make them busier than they need be. It takes a conscious effort to try to cut down on the busyness.

Good to be wanted

Managers may, and often do, grumble at being interrupted by telephone calls and personal callers, yet they enjoy the feeling of being wanted. They may pride themselves on being always available when people want them and so resist suggestions that it can be an inefficient use of their time; it may also be frustrating to their staff because they may get no opportunity for a more thoughtful discussion.

Play areas

Some senior managers, especially those who enjoyed the operational work they did, find the more abstract work of senior management unfulfilling and, at times, long to be more hands-on. They may satisfy this longing by having a play area that is not part of their current job but which they may justify by saying they are particularly good at doing it. They may not be aware they are doing so, although their staff will notice it, particularly if it is part of their job. Play areas may be therapeutic and so justifiable, but the player needs to recognise what he or she is doing and its repercussions on others.

Pleasures of troubleshooting

The more senior the job, the harder it can be to see results from your work, because the job becomes more one of getting things done through other people – one of the definitions of managing. Troubleshooting can provide a rare opportunity to see quick results from your actions, so it is a temptation to enjoy the pleasure of trying to sort out the problem, even though the task may be better left to other people and they may object to not being left to cope and to get their enjoyment, too.

Responding to fashions

It is remarkable that managers are almost as influenced by fashion as dress designers, and there are plenty of consultants making their living by selling the latest management fashion. Like dress designers, similar ideas recur, even if they have different names. The NHS is particularly fashion conscious, as skimming the job titles in recruitments ads over the last few years will show. Fashions have good points: in dress, they make the wearer of the new fashion feel good; in management, they provide a spur for looking again at old problems, but they can also be a distraction and be linked to unnecessary spending on consultants. Research studies of the results of applying the latest management fashion show that doing so often leads to disappointment.

Shaped or shaping?

One of the major differences between effective managers and the others is that effective managers have a clear view of what they are trying to achieve and take every opportunity to move nearer to doing so. All managers have to spend time reacting to the unexpected, but effective managers also have a strategic view, which they keep in mind so they can make good use of unexpected opportunities. John Kotter, who studied 15 general managers, found that when they were in a new job they gradually developed their own agendas.[2] These agendas were less formal than objectives, more fluid and personal as the manager in a new job discovered what particular contributions he or she wished to make and developed personal strategies for doing so. But many managers do not develop their own agendas, or if they do, fail to realise them because they are still swept along by events and by other people's expectations of what they should do.

Managing relationships is an important aspect of achieving your agenda, particularly where, as in the health and social services, there are many, often complex, relationships. There needs to be a strategic view of what the jobholder should be doing about each of the most important relationships; also whether new relationships need to be developed to achieve the strategy.

Making time

Time is both finite and elastic: its elasticity is recognised by the phrase 'if you want something done ask a busy man' (has it been modernised to 'ask a busy person'?). The people who manage to achieve a remarkable amount and range of work do so because they are good at organising their time. That many managers recognise this is something they could do better is shown by the market over the years for expensive short courses and books on managing your time. Some managers benefit from the time-management courses, which may include a special time-management diary, but for others the result is like that of many New Year's resolutions. Even if you are not disciplined enough to use a time-management diary, you may find the following simple guidelines helpful:

- keep a running record of what you do for a week; you may think you know what you are doing, but many managers who keep such diaries are surprised, and often shocked, at what they find. It is evidence of what you are actually doing,[3] and unless you collect such evidence, or get a secretary to do so for you, it is easy to have an inaccurate idea of how you spend your time
- notice particularly whether you are 'a stream-of-consciousness manager', one who does what comes into mind next, thus interrupting yourself. The danger is that this can become such a habit that you cannot settle to a task that really needs your concentrated attention
- if you decide, after keeping a diary, that you have too fragmented a work pattern, ask yourself who you should be available to and how quickly. It is often more efficient

for both boss and subordinate to have a regular time together than to talk with each other whenever they think about it. You could have times when you are known to be available and others when you are known to be working in your office and prefer not to be disturbed. If you also walk around, observing what is going on and talking with your staff, as is customary in some jobs, this can give staff an opportunity to raise queries with you or tell you something you may otherwise not hear

- keep a list of outstanding tasks and tick them off as you do them, but also have a method for picking up those non-urgent tasks you are always postponing
- if you are senior enough to have a secretary, use her to organise your time if you are not good at doing so yourself
- look at someone you know who gets an unusual amount of work done, without working very long hours, and try to discover how they do it.

Attention is a scarce resource

There is too much to do: this is the cry of many managers. However hard they work, there is more they could usefully do. Therefore a common managerial problem is prioritising what to do, which problems to attend to and which opportunities for improvement or new developments to pursue. Some managers do this very carefully, deciding what most needs their attention. Others are more reactive and are carried along by events and their own way of working. The problems most likely to get attention are those where there is an external pressure to deal with them. In the public sector, especially in politically sensitive parts of it, there can be strong pressure to deal with particular kinds of problem, such as the length of NHS waiting lists. The danger is that attention may be focused on these, and the wider aims and perspectives are forgotten.

Managers who want to practise evidence-based management should ensure that they and their team are getting the evidence they need to help them decide which of the problems and opportunities they should be examining, apart from the political imperatives. One guideline is to have a sufficiently good monitoring system to give warning of problems or potential problems: this is so important that it is discussed further in Chapter 4. Another guideline is to check whether enough attention is being paid to the different stakeholders. What managers choose to attend to, where there is a choice, is a key determinant of effective management, but one that has received surprisingly little attention. Noordegraaf, who studied public managers in Holland, points out that: 'Attention is the prime managerial resource, but it is the scarcest as well'.[4]

This suggests that another useful way of recording what you actually do is to note over the course of a week what you gave most attention to each day, and whether this was in line with what you think it is most important for you to do in the job. If you decide that particular events blew you off course, do the same for another week and see how the two compare. This may tell you whether the first week was unusual and, if not, what you can and should do to manage the job better.

Making space

Many managers think there are so many demands on them that they have no time to think strategically about what they should be doing or to do many of the things they think are important. A simple model (Figure 2.1) shows why this view is likely to be wrong. The author developed the model to explain why her research showed that managers in similar jobs do them so differently.[5] The figure illustrates the amount of freedom that exists in managerial and clinical jobs for the jobholder to do the job in a distinctive way not just in *how* it

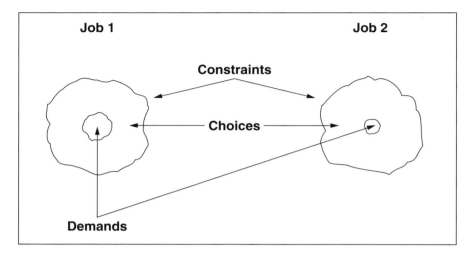

Figure 2.1   Model of a managerial job.

is done, the managerial or clinical style, but more importantly in *what* is done.

The figure shows an inner core of the job, the demands. These are the work things anyone in the past would have to do to be considered adequate in the job. The outer boundary is the constraints: these are all the factors that restrict what the jobholder can do, such as resources, space, regulations, deadlines, and the abilities and attitudes of staff, colleagues and boss. In between demands and constraints is an area labelled 'choices': these are the opportunities in the job for one jobholder to do different work from another. The lines in the diagram are wavy to show that each is subject to change, from changes in the situation or by actions of the jobholder. Constraints, for example, can and do change: the boss changes and the new one has different expectations of what the jobholder must do; the jobholder is successful in over-coming some of the constraints, thus creating more choice; changes in regulations or resources may reduce or increase the constraints. Jobs differ too, which is why the figure shows two jobs. Some jobs offer more choice than others and cover a larger area, but all managerial jobs, and most others too, offer some choice – that of emphasising some aspects of the job more than others and seeking to reduce the constraints.

The model, which has been used by many managers, can help you to take a more realistic look at the demands and constraints and recognise that there are more choices than you thought. Where there is a choice, there should be a strategy to help you decide how to make best use of it or whether to ignore that choice and concentrate on another aspect of the job. Often managers find that what they had considered to be demands are, in part, self-imposed, so really a choice. A strategic view will include re-examining such self-imposed demands and asking how important they are. It should also ask what demands and/or constraints the individual can seek to influence or change: these can include trying to shape the expectations of other people, including the boss, about what the jobholder should be doing.

Individuals differ in their approach to constraints. Some see them as givens, some may even welcome them because they reduce uncertainty and the need to act, while others regard them as an obstacle to be circumvented where possible. Many of the demands and constraints on managers are imposed by the expectations of those with whom they work, and these are not set forever. Managers can seek to influence them: this is one of their choices.

Managers differ in their capacity to analyse their jobs. Some can describe it from the outside, in an objective way. Others think of the job as being part of themselves, believing that they have so moulded the job that it cannot be described as separate from themselves. Managers who want to take a strategic view of their job must be able to look at the job objectively and to assess their own abilities, ambitions and inclinations to decide what they want to achieve in the job and how to go about doing so.

If you observe how two managers or two clinicians in similar posts do their jobs, you can witness the choices an individual takes and then seek to apply this way of thinking to your own situation. Look, for example, at how much time they spend with different people: some managers, for example, spend much longer with members of their staff than others; some spend much more time cultivating external contacts. They also differ in what they spend that time doing; for example, some managers will spend time coaching their staff, while others may make more use of them as a source of information about what is happening. Considering how other people do their jobs can make it easier to apply the same thinking to your own job; you should look at *what* they do, as well as *how* they do it. However, we more commonly notice how people work, rather than thinking about what they do. Practise analysing the latter by looking at your colleagues, or at the differences between teachers of a management programme or between different bosses you have had. An important choice is the area of the job in which the manager is trying to have an impact. Again, observing other managers can show how widely this can differ.

It is only possible to find time to practise evidence-based management if you make the space to do so. One way of achieving this is to use the demands, constraints and choices model as a way of recognising that there are choices in your job and that you need to take a strategic view of these choices. Understanding how you work and reviewing whether you could work more effectively is another way of making space.

Beliefs about managing

A belief is an acceptance of something as true or real that is not a demonstrable fact. We all have beliefs, even if we do not believe in a god. These include beliefs about managing. This fact receives little attention since the language used for talking about management is formal and general, using words like 'objectives', 'performance criteria' and 'planning'. Yet when managers are interviewed about their work they often want to describe their beliefs about how to manage. Tony Watson, who was a participant observer in a factory, gives a vivid account of such beliefs in *In Search of Management*.[6] Managers' beliefs structure how they see their job and determine how they tackle it. One manager may believe that the most important thing to do is to please the boss; another that building a good team matters most, another that walking around and chatting to staff is the key to knowing what is happening, while another manager may attach more importance to performance figures, and yet another believes that understanding the politics of the organisation is essential for making changes and for making career progress. Then there are beliefs about how you manage: some managers believe that managing is mainly intuitive, whereas others think it is more of a science and that you must learn the tools of management. Many may hold these views with conviction. **The beliefs managers hold will influence whether they will accept the need for, even the possibility of, evidence-based management.** Understanding and questioning your own beliefs about managing, and those with whom you work, is one aspect of a strategy for encouraging and practising evidence-based management.

Understanding your strengths and weaknesses

In addition to the common lessons described about how to manage the job, individuals have their own strengths and weaknesses which should be taken into account. The relevance of this to practising evidence-based management is discussed later; what is important here is to remember that in thinking about how to manage your job better – if you need to do this – you should be realistic about what you do well and what you do not.

Summary

To practise evidence-based management you have to be on top of your job, otherwise you will be too harassed to be able to do so. You have to manage your time well and suggestions are made for ways of doing so. Keeping a record of what you do each day for at least a week is a good way of checking on how you actually spend your time. You should be aware of, and try not to yield to, the seductions of management. The most tempting ones for many managers are:

- enjoying being busy and feeling indispensable
- indulging in play areas
- eager involvement in troubleshooting
- responding too uncritically to the latest management fashion.

You need to recognise that attention is a prime, but scarce, managerial resource and one that should be allocated thoughtfully. Your beliefs about managing will help to determine your attitude to evidence-based management.

You need to find space in your job so that you can think and act strategically. A simple model developed from the author's research, comparing the work of managers in similar jobs, shows that all jobs offer choice in what work is done as well as in how it is done. The research also shows that these choices may go unrecognised. It is easy to exaggerate the core of demands, that is, work that must be done, and the constraints that limit what can be done. If you think strategically you will recognise the choices that exist and consider where you can best make your contribution. You will seek, where necessary, to reduce the constraints and to shape people's expectations of what you should be doing.

References

1   Carlson S (1951 and 1991) *Executive Behaviour: reprinted with contributions by Henry Mintzberg and Rosemary Stewart.* Acta Universitatis Uppsaliensis, Uppsala.
2   Kotter J (1982) *The General Managers.* The Free Press, New York.
3   Stewart R (1988) *Managers and their Jobs: a study of the similarities and differences in the ways managers spend their time* (2e). Macmillan, Basingstoke. This gives examples of different kinds of diary, either to look at the work as a whole or at particular aspects of it.
4   Noordegraaf M (2000) *Attention! Work and Behavior of Public Managers Amidst Ambiguity.* Eburon, Delft, p. 86.
5   Stewart R (1982) *Choices for the Manager: a guide to managerial work and behaviour.* McGraw-Hill, London.
6   Watson TJ (2001) (revised) *In Search of Management: culture, chaos and control in managerial work.* Thomson Learning, London.

3

Using information and knowledge

A manager is a craftsperson whose raw material is information.[1]

Clinicians do not, I think, regard management as a skill with an associated evidence base. When one starts to use techniques that are more grounded in theory it is interesting to watch other professionals' changing attitudes.
Senior nurse manager

A craftsperson should understand the nature of the material with which he or she works and be skilful in his or her use of it. This chapter seeks to help managers, and clinicians in their managerial role, to understand the nature of the information with which they work and to improve their knowledge and skill in doing so. Unless that is done, evidence-based management cannot be practised successfully.

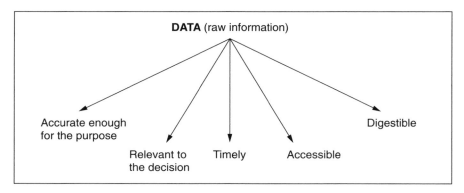

Figure 3.1   Requirements of good information.

Requirements for good information

Figure 3.1 illustrates what is required to get good information. It starts with 'data', which are the raw material for information, and shows what is needed before the data can be
useful information. Data need to be accurate, but only accurate enough for the purpose. Sometimes precise data are
required, but often managers need only the best information
available within the time limit for the decision making. Often
decisions have to be made before there is enough information
to be confident that it is the right decision, and you should be
alert to possible inadequacies in the information when
checking on how the decision is working out.

The information has to be timely, particularly if a decision
is needed quickly. Usually it should also be easily accessible
and digestible by those wanting to use it. Sometimes esoteric
information, which is hard to get and hard to understand,
may also be needed.

The information has to be relevant to the subject, which
may not be easy to judge. There are two possible dangers:
one, that the subject may not have been adequately under-
stood; and two, that the information may not really be what
is needed. For example, an increased labour turnover among

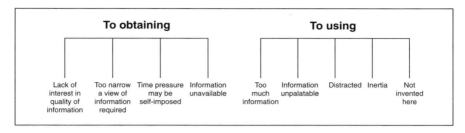

Figure 3.2   Obstacles to obtaining and using information.

specialist staff may be causing anxiety. This may be thought to be due to the lower rewards being given than by those who are competing for the same staff, so up-to-date information is collected about this. However, there are many other possible reasons for high specialist turnover, so collecting information about why people are leaving may be more relevant.

Obstacles to obtaining and using information

Evidence-based management is about finding the information required and then using it. This sounds logical, but there are a number of reasons why this may not happen; these are shown in Figure 3.2.

Caring about the quality of information being used is an essential part of practising evidence-based management. The case study from Frimley Park given later in the chapter is a good example of a careful approach to thinking about what information is relevant and ensuring its accuracy.

A common reason for not getting the right information is having too narrow a view of what you need to know. The scale of the subject may be underestimated, as may its complexity. For example, when evaluating outcomes of change it is easy to forget how difficult it can be to distinguish cause and effect. If, for example, you are trying to assess the value of a management training programme, it is hard to distinguish the possible effects of the programme on managerial performance from the other factors that may have influenced it.

A major reason why the information received may be inadequate or wrong is that those giving it think that accurate information, if it is unfavourable, will count against them. If you doubt that this is true, think of the occasions when you were economical with the truth because you wanted to conceal particular problems that you or your unit were having. To try and limit the amount of misinformation you receive, either deliberately or by mistake, cultivate a wide range of contacts. Walking around rather than staying in the office can also make it easier to pick up useful information, like the new chief executive who was told when she was doing so: 'You look honest, so let me tell you about the financial scams that are going on here'.

The way you react to staff who do try to tell you about problems will affect what you are told next time. Some managers do not want to hear bad news; some may even treat the bearer of bad news as if they were the problem, as many whistle-blowers have found. Some of the scandals identified by the Commission for Health Improvement (CHI) in 2000 suggest that a useful guide in the health service is: 'Listen to the concerns of nurses', since these could have prevented the continuation of some medical scandals.

The lack of availability of information required is a real obstacle, although individuals will vary in how good they are at getting information. Some have, and make use of, a much wider network of contacts; some are much better than others at knowing where and how to look for information. Individuals differ, too, in how much importance they attach to getting good information and hence in how easily they conclude that they cannot get it. But beware using the need for more information as an excuse to postpone taking a decision!

The obstacles to using information vary with the type and character of the organisation. The danger of being over-whelmed with information can be greater in the public sector, because so many instructions, advice and other information may come from the government. The strength of the other four obstacles shown in Figure 3.2 will vary with the reactions of the individual manager and of the group. The information may be considered too unpalatable to use as a basis for action, and hence be ignored, either because it does not support the decision the individual or group wishes to reach or because the consequences of acting on the information are too frightening: a reaction to some of the investigations of disasters. Another, and often appropriate, reason for not acting on the information is that more pressing problems, or better opportunities, intervene.

Inertia can be a serious obstacle to using information for decisions in some organisations, particularly in those that do not have a dynamic culture. Although all may agree the information shows that a change is needed, there is not sufficient momentum for anything to happen. The last obstacle shown in Figure 3.2 is 'not invented here'; some may prefer to work out their own solution rather than consider how other people have dealt with similar problems. This may be a greater problem in the public sector than in companies where the competitive pressure can be a spur to taking up others' successful practice. This suggests that in the annual Health Management Awards of the *Health Service Journal* there should be a category for applying other people's successes!

Human limitations in reasoning

This is the source of a quite different obstacle to the effective use of information. Research has taught us a lot about how people think and about how they interpret the world around them. It tells us that people are not reasoning machines: they have their personal ways of seeing and interpreting what is happening. Two people in the same situation can behave differently because they see it differently. One person, for example, may see it as an opportunity, another as a threat.

We all have our own mental maps that help us interpret the world around us. So our view of reality may differ from somebody else's and we may have to negotiate about whose view of reality is to be accepted. But first we have to recognise that there can be genuine differences in how people see a situation.

Research has also found that people have common limitations in their reasoning capacity and to offset these use a simplified model to deal with a complex problem. We have to simplify if we are to survive. There are also common biases in the use of information, as distinct from the biases that come from an individual's personality, background and position. Research shows that there are four common ways in which people are biased in their selection and use of information.

- *By starting from an anchor point in making judgements.* For example, in deciding whether a man is tall, one must have a view of what is average height. In thinking about what further information you need you will tend to start from the information that is currently available.
- *Decision makers tend to use only the available information in the form it is presented.* This means there can be a danger that they are too dependent on the ability and interest of the presenter to provide the most relevant and timely information – a useful warning for many groups making decisions, particularly those in formal groups like boards of directors.
- *Recent events are given more importance than earlier ones.*
- *Not thinking about probabilities,* so that undue importance may be given to a few occurrences and if two things occur simultaneously thinking that one must have caused the other.

The first point can be illustrated by how a manager interprets the performance of two staff members, one of whom he judges to be a good performer and the other a poor one. A positive feeling about a subordinate can be the anchor point for making judgements, predisposing the manager to look for indications of good performance and to evaluate him or her more favourably than is deserved; there can be the reverse for someone the manager does not like.

Psychological researchers have identified many other ways in which people are biased in how they use information. These include:

- seeking information that is consistent with the cultural norms of the organisation
- giving more weight to concrete information and less to more ambiguous and subjective information
- inconsistency of judgements, e.g. in selection criteria
- conservatism: failing to revise opinions when new information appears
- first and sometimes last items in the presentation of data can get undue importance
- assuming a linear development of a trend, whereas it may be exponential, as in an epidemic
- selecting data to support a particular argument rather than looking for data that might refute it
- unjustified optimism.

An overall warning about human limitations in reasoning comes in a book about the inferences people mistakenly make:

> *Epistemologists from Bacon to Russell are agreed on a fundamental and pervasive human failing ... the tendency toward overconfidence in one's judgments, towards greater certainty about one's assessments, theories, and conclusions than closely reasoned analysis*

could possibly justify.... If people have a clearer notion about the kinds of judgments and inferences that are likely to show error, perhaps their ill-founded certainty might be shaken.[2]

The listing above of some of the more common human failings in reasoning helps show where you should be on your guard against overconfidence in your judgements, and thus improve your practice of evidence-based management.

Sources of information

One way of trying to improve your use of information is to examine the different sources, consider whether appropriate use is being made of each and explore whether more should be done to improve what is obtained from each source. There are five main sources of information:

- the organisational systems established to monitor what is happening: these may be created by the individual manager or the group, inherited or passed down from above
- the written sources of information, whether on paper or on the Web
- people within or outside the organisation, who may volunteer information or who can be approached for help
- the manager's experience
- the values of the organisation, which influence what people look for and how they look.

Organisational monitoring systems

Organisational monitoring systems are so important an aspect of evidence-based management that they are the subject of Chapter 4.

Written sources of information

'Written' now has to be used very broadly as it can range from traditional books and journals, available in libraries or personally owned or borrowed, to information on the Web. Increasingly, some information, including certain journals and books, is only available on the Web or downloaded from it. On balance, this makes it easier to practise evidence-based management because a wide range of information is available very quickly. However, there is more opportunity for inaccurate information to be provided on the Web than in the more reputable journals, because it may not have gone through any vetting procedure. There are numerous useful digests of information in print and on the Web, with many newspapers running pieces on useful information sites on the Web. Evidence-based managers should know which are the most relevant digests for them.

It is helpful to have an understanding of what research has told us about behaviour in organisations as it can be a useful guide to reorganisation and to developing human relations policies, particularly for the management of change. One common change that affects many different kinds of organisations is mergers, yet too often the lessons of research into the handling of mergers are either unknown or ignored.

West Berkshire Community Trust is an example of the use made of research on the experience of mergers and acquisitions in the private sector. Two of the lessons from this work were used as a guide to handling a merger between the West Berkshire Priority Care Service NHS Trust and East Berkshire Learning Disability Trust. The first lesson, which has been shown in many research studies, is that one should 'communicate, communicate' because of people's level of anxiety, even when there is nothing new to say. Different communication media should also be used, because anxious people may not take in what is being said if it is only said once or only one medium is used. The trust introduced a monthly newsletter, 'Changing Times'. Other methods of communication included regular staff briefings about what was happening, feedback forms and staff conferences. The other lesson taken from experience in the private sector was the importance of 'good endings'.[3]

Some managers neglect research information, perhaps because they have not been trained to use it. If so, there is a choice: get the relevant training and/or try to make sure that you work with, or at least can draw upon, those who do understand what research is relevant.

People as sources of information

Since studies of managerial work show that managers spend a large proportion of their time with other people, it is they who are likely to be the main source of current information. This is true even in large government bureaucracies, especially when there is much change. Good managers, as many studies have shown, cultivate a wide range of contacts with whom they exchange information. John Kotter's study of 15 general managers in American companies[4] found that they spent time refreshing their relations with a large network of useful, and potentially useful, contacts. There are some managerial jobs that depend less on contacts to get the information to do the job effectively, but they are rare and likely to be highly specialist ones. Managers also depend on their staff for the information they need to do their job. We saw above how important it is to try to ensure that your staff give you honest information and are ready to alert you to problems.

E-mail makes it much easier to exchange information and to widen the number and range of people with whom you do so, as you are no longer dependent on the people you have met or others recommend. But for some managers, the volume of e-mail can be daunting and they may wonder whether it is more of a curse than a boon.

People are also a source of research information since much social research is based on asking people their views, often to assess the response to particular policies. This is the primary source of information for appraisal of training programmes and one that is commonly used in pilot programmes and as a way of checking on the response to ongoing programmes. London Ambulance Service NHS Trust provides an example.

Box 3.1: Training of team leaders in London Ambulance

This case study is included because it shows the care taken in designing, piloting and evaluating the effectiveness of a training programme as an aspect of the creation of a new post, that of team leader.

Background
A decision was made to promote 161 paramedic staff between August 2000 and March 2002 to team leader positions with a training officer for each complex to provide clinical leadership and support for individual team leaders. The 'prime responsibilities of the team leader will be to assist in the delivery of high quality patient care; provide leadership and support primarily to a team of operational A&E staff and to act as role model for all staff, fostering high professional standards and encouraging best practice'.* A key function is to monitor and raise operational clinical and non-clinical standards, so it is seen as an important new post, requiring careful planning, piloting and evaluation.
  The first group of team leaders who were appointed, after careful selection, had a two-and-a-half-week non-residential training course before taking up their duties. This group was seen as a pilot to be carefully evaluated before the next group was appointed and trained.

Pilot and evaluation
The team leader pilot, including the training programme, was

evaluated: 'extensive feedback was sought from across the Service to understand what went well, what didn't go quite so well and what lessons could be learnt'. A factual evaluation report was prepared containing over 50 recommendations. This was widely circulated throughout the Service and the feedback considered by the Team Leader Strategy Group in producing the plan for future appointments and training of team leaders; additional information was a risk assessment of possible outcomes during the roll-out process.

Subsequent action
The second training programme was extended from two-and-a-half weeks to five weeks, including a residential week. Comments and feedback were collated from all those involved. The students' assessment was in the form of a rating scale for the extent to which each session met their training needs and comments on each session. They were also asked for additional comments after they returned to their new roles. The results of the student rating were clearly presented in bar diagrams. Comments were also collected from the course director, the key contributors to the programme and the consultants used for the design and delivery of the residential week.

Further changes were made to the training programme as a result of the evaluation. The revised programme was given to two groups in early February 2001. The evaluation of these two programmes will be taken into account in finalising the programme although to ensure consistency across the Service no major changes will be made.

Feedback from team leaders already in post showed the need for a one-day training session to cover areas of the role that had not been foreseen as requiring additional training, such as reports on and from the scene by team leaders. This new training session is being developed by a multidisciplinary team. It will be piloted in two sectors among current team leaders, evaluated and then included in the wider training programme.

---

*London Ambulance Service NHS Trust (Dec 2000) *Team Leader Implementation Pack*.

The manager's own experience

This is a powerful guide for many managers in many situations. Any experienced manager in charge of a process, whether for producing cars, teaching children or treating patients, will have learnt to tell when things are not going well by looking around. This can often provide faster information than any formal monitoring system. An experienced manager will also have learnt whose information can be relied on. It is the personal, intimate knowledge of the activity and of the people that helps managers judge the problems that need attention, but how they decide what most requires their attention will depend on what they really value.

Values of the organisation

In their huge best seller of 20 years ago, *In Search of Excellence*,[5] Peters and Waterman highlighted the importance for successful performance of a well-defined set of guiding beliefs. In doing so, they were not saying anything new, complained envious academics. Such beliefs act as guidelines for action and help to determine what people treat as important and what they look for. Customer satisfaction is important for competitive organisations, so managers are likely to stress this as an organisation value. There is not the same imperative to make client satisfaction a value in the public and voluntary sectors, although governments may try to stress its importance.

How staff are treated will be influenced by cultural beliefs about the importance and rights of staff. Some companies treat their staff much better than the public sector, especially the NHS, has done. In some companies, the strength of beliefs about the good treatment of customers and/or staff can be traced back to the strong beliefs of the founders of the firm. The

American IT company Hewlett Packard is a good example, as are the early Quaker firms like Cadbury and Rowntree.

Visiting companies with strong beliefs about customer and employee satisfaction can help to alert you to what values are considered important there and what gets measured as a result. There can also be considerable differences between similar kinds of organisation in the values that are treated as important, so visits to an organisation like yours can reveal different values in practice.

Organising information for yourself

In the public services, more information is written down, whether on paper or on screen, than in the private sector. There is often a surfeit of information, making it difficult to keep up to date with the flow and easy to fail to read something that requires action. The problem for the manager, especially managers in the public sector, is what to attend to. It helps to work out what information you are most likely to need and what are the best ways of trying to ensure you get it. Drucker, in *Management Challenges for the 21st Century*,[6] suggests some methods of doing so.

- *Key events* – which are the key ones by which my performance will be judged? Key events in a politically sensitive organisation such as the NHS will include areas that politicians think the public will judge them by. Getting waiting lists down has been a key event under both Conservative and Labour governments. In public companies, key events are usually linked to the reporting of income and expenditure, an analysis of sales and the progress of particular initiatives.
- *Abnormal fluctuations* – each manager has to decide which are the key figures to be monitored and know the normal fluctuations and the abnormal ones that call for action. This may be hard sometimes so it can be useful to hold periodic

management meetings to discuss the unusual events that have occurred in each person's area of responsibility. Individually these may not seem significant, but there may be a pattern that requires attention.

- *Threshold concept* – deciding at what level a number of events becomes a trend requiring action, for example when a disease becomes an epidemic or the number of resignations rises. The threshold for life-threatening incidents, whether in dangerous plants or in healthcare, can be one spectacular incident that causes multiple loss of life or injury. Spectacular events, like Dr Harold Shipman murdering his patients, are a trigger for investigating failures in systems that should be protecting patients.

Knowing how to find the best sources of information is a useful skill for managers who want to practise evidence-based management. This is easier today with the growth of IT and the increasing number of information management specialists with the task of ensuring good and readily accessible information. Yet many managers still prefer to turn to other people, either by phone or e-mail, when they want to know what is happening. Reluctantly, sometimes, information specialists have had to accept the popularity of such informal information and even to facilitate it via the Internet, so that those who are good gatekeepers of information can be known outside their own circle.

Taking a broad view

It is important to make good use of the different sources of information, but it may also be important to look at the process or problem as a whole. The case in Box 3.2 illustrates both the care taken to get accurate data and the capacity to look at the task as a whole and consider what different aspects are relevant.

Box 3.2:   Implementing the two-week cancer appointments in Frimley Park Hospital

The case is included for the following reasons:
- it is an example of care taken to ensure accurate data, identification of different ways in which the data may be inaccurate, including how particular codes are used in practice, and the recognition of the need to consider future coding needs
- it illustrates the ability to see the process as a whole rather than focusing on only one aspect of it, hence showing the different kinds of information needed. There is a parallel here with the use of industrial engineers in manufacturing companies to examine a process and consider ways in which it can be improved.

Background
The White Paper **The New NHS** included the following pledge for reducing waiting times for cancer patients:

Everyone with a suspected cancer will be able to see a specialist within two weeks of their GP deciding that they need to be seen urgently and requesting an appointment. By April 1999 for breast cancer and by 2000 for all other cancers.

The specifics of implementation were spelt out later. The waiting times for a consultant's appointment for suspected breast cancer were to be monitored from 1 April 1999 by a new return (QMCW). New National Guidelines (March 2000) said that it is the GP who decides whether a patient needs to be seen urgently and requires a specialist outpatient appointment within two weeks. Every referral made under the two-week rule had to be clearly identified as urgent and include the date of the decision to refer. A referral had to be received by the trust within 24 hours of that date. This became a requirement in the summer of 1999. The definitive guidelines were published on the Internet in March 2000 (due for review in 2001).

How Frimley Park Hospital tackled meeting the new standard
In Frimley Park Hospital, a Cancer Unit Steering Group was established in the early autumn of 1999. The Group decided that the way to meet this target was to make it the responsibility of one person, a nurse whom the doctors could trust to sift the referrals to see if they met the guidelines set out in the circular. Because Frimley Park was the first hospital in their area (South East Region) to decide how to meet the new requirement they could not draw on others' experience; anyway, the required speed of implementation meant that all must decide quickly what to do.

The Cancer Unit Co-ordinator, Steph Thorns, was appointed on 1 April 2000. Her main duty is to report on the hospital's record in meeting the two-week target and seek to ensure that appointments are made within that time. She sees her tasks to be:

- to ensure that the coding data are accurate. She found that they were not appropriate for monitoring the new standard. She took the following actions to improve data relevance and accuracy and to consider the implications of the coding for the breakdown of cancer type for future returns:
  - she discovered that some non-urgent patients had been added where there were spaces left in a clinic but had been classified as TWR (two-week referral) because that was the only 'appointment type' available
  - to get the pre-registration department to use PAS (Patient Administration System) to include the date of referral on the registration page so that reports can be generated later
  - to ensure that the coding system would assist in the breakdown of cancer types for future returns
- to ensure that all urgent referrals are picked up:
  - to encourage GPs to send their urgent referrals by fax to the TWR office, but also to ensure that they are picked up however they arrive – some go to consultants' fax machines and some come in by letter. She now asks the pre-registration department to tell her of all letters marked TWR and she can then remind the practice that they should have used the central fax

   – to use a TWR stamp and date stamp to highlight the urgent
     referral letters
- to ensure use of the available consultant capacity by encouraging
  GPs to refer generically rather than to a specific consultant, and
  to get consultants' agreement that she can make the booking
  with the relevant specialist
- to streamline the appointments system by booking the breast
  cancer appointments herself and making sure that the necessary
  investigations are done on the same day before the consultant's
  appointment. She has arranged for time slots to be available in
  the X-ray department so that the mammograms can be done
  before the appointment. She has also changed the system to take
  account of this so that patients receive just one letter about their
  appointment. She ensures that the same is done for the other
  cancer clinics
- to identify how many patients are referred by GPs with a two-
  week flag on them.

Methods of evaluation
The main evaluation is that all patients whom the GPs say need an
urgent appointment are seen within two weeks.

   Monitoring of all urgent cancer referrals in November 2000
showed that there were 129 two-week cancer referrals of which all
but one were seen within two weeks, and for that one there had
been a delay of eight days in the referral arriving, but the patient
was then seen within two weeks.

   In February 2001, a detailed analysis by type of cancer was
made of all cancer two-week referrals. This showed 100% achievement for all those attending during February, including those
whose referrals had not been received within 24 hours.

   Other benefits of the new system in Frimley Park are streamlining
of the process of testing and examining the patient so that it all
takes places on the same day, and better utilisation of clinics as, in
addition to the clinical staff monitoring appointments usage, the
Cancer Unit Co-ordinator can fill up slots at short notice,
contacting patients directly.

   Steph Thorns has identified other ways in which the process of
handling appointments for urgent cancers might be improved, and

reports will be produced on:
- number of referrals who were subsequently found to have cancer
- number of cancers that were not referred urgently and their referral source
- an audit of referral letters
- referral patterns by GPs/primary care groups.

The design of an executive training programme provides a quite different example of the merit of taking a broad view of the information needed. There are the obvious questions that most programme designers would ask, such as: Who is the programme for? What are its aims? How should success be judged? Other questions that could usefully be asked include:

- What can participants be expected to know already?
- Is their level of knowledge likely to differ much?
- If so, should account be taken of this?
- Does participants' attention vary at different times of the day or different periods of the course?
- If so, what account needs to be taken of this in designing the programme?
- Are senior managers going to visit?
- If so, how can best use be made of their presence?

Such questions can help in designing a programme and in considering how to appraise it.

Knowledge and its management

Knowledge is a broader term than information. It includes the knowledge available about a subject, such as human resource management or the treatment of diabetes. Knowledge is both academic and practical: there is the knowledge taught for an

MBA about human behaviour and there is the individual's own acquired knowledge about how to treat people to encourage them to do what is wanted. People use their knowledge to check the information they receive and to determine its value.

Sometimes the words 'information' and 'knowledge' are used interchangeably: the Institute of Health Sciences in Oxford has used 'knowledge' rather than 'information' in advocating an 'International Knowledge Partnership Health and Environment' to promote evidence-based decision making. They advocate a five-stage plan for better knowledge management for international health and population.

1 Knowledge production – producing the knowledge that decision makers need.
2 Knowledge storage – making the knowledge available.
3 Knowledge appraisal – determining its quality and relevance.
4 Knowledge implementation – getting research into practice.
5 Knowledge marketing – forming public–private partnerships to disseminate knowledge.[7]

This is a very formal view of knowledge. It is one aspect of knowledge and the aspect that is much easier to capture and store. But an important aspect of individuals' knowledge is tacit: the skills they have learnt. Some of this can be taught to others, as many medical and nursing skills can be taught, but some knowledge remains too individual and instinctive – the developed instinct of experience – to be formally taught. However, it is possible to learn by watching how good managers or good clinicians go about their work, observing the way they react to situations and people. In our enthusiasm for knowledge capture, storage and dissemination it is important to remember the importance of tacit knowledge.

Knowledge but no action

This is depressingly common: it often takes a long time to get new knowledge adopted. Such delay is an old problem, as Locke said:

Truth scarce ever yet carried it by vote anywhere at its first appearance.

Several medical studies have shown that it takes up to ten years for even very strong evidence of the value of a treatment to become established practice.[8] The famous late nineteenth- and early-twentieth century doctor, William Osler, delivering the Harveian Oration at the Royal College of Physicians of London in 1906 on 'The growth of truth, as illustrated in the discovery of the circulation of the blood', said:

We may have become more plastic and receptive, but I doubt it; even our generation – that great generation of the last quarter of the nineteenth century – had a practical demonstration of the slowness of the acceptation of an obvious truth in the long fight for the aseptic treatment of wounds.... [It was] a long and grievous battle, as many of us well know who had to contend in hospitals with the opposition of men who could not – not who would not – see the truth.[9]

If in medicine, where the evidence is so much stronger than it is ever likely to be in management, there is a long delay in the take-up of good new ideas, then the response to information initiatives like Beacons* may be disappointing. What is needed

---

* Beacons is a generic term used for schemes in government which acknowledge sites of good practice that then participate in dissemination activities to spread their good practice. In 2001, there were Beacon

to judge their effects is evidence about what changes have actually been made as a result of learning from the Beacon site. Such evidence can only be indicative rather than certain, because of the difficulties of being sure about cause and effect: even if similar changes are made in an organisation that has had contact with the Beacon site there may have been other factors that resulted in, or contributed to, the change.

We should have learnt from the long history of the difficulties in getting new ideas adopted that a necessary subject for research is how to do this. There is research on the diffusion of innovation,[10] but this mainly remains in the academic world and has not had much effect in the world of public policy. As Nutley and Davies point out:

> *It remains an irony that so many of the activities surrounding evidence-based practice are not in themselves evidence based. While the existing literature in several fields can offer guidance and insight, there is as yet only a limited empirical base evaluating specific evidence-based strategies.*[11]

They go on to suggest areas for research on the implementation of evidence-based practice.

Inertia was mentioned earlier as a serious problem in organisations: it affects the application of knowledge and the implementation of decisions. Two Harvard professors have written a book about it, called *The Knowing–Doing Gap: how*

---

schemes in schools, police, local government and central government. The NHS Beacon programme was initiated as part of the 2000 NHS Plan. Each year organisations that are an example of good practice in particular subjects, such as mental health or human resources, are selected as Beacons and given a grant to enable them to make their experience available to others. Information about a particular Beacon can be found in the annual *NHS Beacons Learning Handbook* and from the website; this includes the name of a contact person and how to access them. Workshops and visits are organised as learning activities.

smart companies turn knowledge into actions.[12] They point out how remarkable it is that there are so few changes in what organisations actually do, despite all the management education and training, consulting and research, as well as all the books and articles. They suggest that one of the reasons is that managers want to learn how to do something rather than the philosophy behind the doing. They urge companies – but the advice applies to the public sector too – to measure their knowing–doing gap and then do something about it.

There can also be a major problem of inertia about using knowledge to tackle long-standing problems such as the time spent waiting for an outpatient appointment and the time spent waiting in the clinic. Is it that these widespread problems in the NHS are intractable ones? Is that the reason why they are of such long standing? Or is it, at least in part, because it is easier to think that the very real difficulties of staff shortages, increasing demand and inadequate facilities make the problems insuperable? Perhaps the will is lacking to tackle the difficulties of change. Yet there is evidence, old and new, that improvements can be made. One example of really old evidence, but still likely to be true today, is a 1965 Nuffield Provincial Hospitals Trust (now called the Nuffield Trust) study on 'Waiting in Outpatient Departments: a survey of out-patient appointments systems', which showed that the two major causes of waiting appeared to be the lateness of doctors and the poor design of appointment systems. Both defects could be remedied, or at least reduced, without spending more money. The government's latest drive to reduce waiting time for appointments has provided a new impetus to tackle the problem.

Knowledge management

Knowledge management is a new specialty in organisations, particularly companies: it is a development in thinking about the nature of information and how to manage it. It recognises that knowledge is in people's heads as well as in records and that sometimes it may only be in their heads, It seeks to make use of the intellectual capital of knowledge organisations – those whose main product is ideas rather than goods – by adding to information management ideas drawn from human resource management and from change management about how to facilitate the sharing of knowledge.

The current fashion for knowledge management exists mainly in the private sector. It started from the concern that firms in knowledge industries, such as consulting, must manage and protect their knowledge base. The departure of key staff in merchant banking, for example, showed that much of the firm's capital was in its employees' heads and not recorded or shared. But even in the public services, good management of knowledge within the organisation is important, particularly in sharing of know-how in dealing with particular problems.

One problem with the aim of capturing the knowledge in employees' heads is who owns the knowledge? Is it the employer's or the individual's? There is a conflict of interest as the organisation wants to encode and share knowledge so as to improve efficiency, but the individual may want to keep their knowledge private as a career asset. This is much more of a problem in companies than in the public sector, where professional staff are more likely to be willing to share knowledge for the common good. The organisation's culture will determine whether knowledge hoarding is common.

Unshared knowledge is one of the problems identified by knowledge management scholars.[13] A useful area to check is whether there is good knowledge sharing between managers and the staff who work for them. Managers can do this by asking their staff what information they need from them. But they should also be ready to answer the same question from their staff. To do this they need to think carefully about the information they need and about the information that would be useful to their staff, but also to be receptive if their staff suggest other information that they need. People at different levels in a hierarchy have access to information, particularly unrecorded information, that is not accessible to those at a different level. It is that information particularly that may be valuable to those at a more junior or a more senior level. The exchange of information between managers and their staff is often inadequate, sometimes because neither thinks about what information the other needs, and sometimes because staff are afraid to tell their boss unwelcome news.

Another area to check is whether there is sufficient knowledge sharing in newly formed work groups, particularly short-term ones where it is important to understand quickly what the different members can contribute. It should be one of the tasks of the leader or chair of the group to make sure he or she knows enough about the members' background to call upon those who are most likely to be able to contribute. He or she should also ensure that, at the first meeting, members learn enough about the other people's background to recognise what distinctive contribution they could make.

The early information management specialists had a very formal view of organisation, believing that if the right technology was installed it would have the intended effects on the way the organisation works. The many disappointments with new IT systems were one of the reasons for the development of knowledge management and of the ideas behind it that emphasise tacit knowledge. Now, one can find IT specialists warning of the danger of overlooking this knowledge and of failing to realise the costs of abandoning the old and learning the new.[14]

'Imagination is more important than knowledge'?

If this was an exam question, one could add 'discuss' to make a challenging question. The query has been added to the quote from Gareth Morgan's *Imaginisation: the art of creative management.*[15] In this, he quotes Einstein:

> *To raise new questions, new possibilities, to regard old problems from a new angle requires creative imagination and marks real advance in science.*

Morgan points out the danger of seeing knowledge as objective or literal truth when all knowledge is the result of interpretation. Different people may place different interpretations on it, and these can change over time as we gain a new perspective. In Chapter 1, we saw that the different interpretations put on evidence are one of the reasons for the controversy that can surround evidence-based medicine. Morgan suggests that one should not look for an authoritative interpretation of a situation, but rather use what he calls 'imaginisation' to realise that any situation can have many dimensions and meanings depending on how the situation is interpreted. What we need, he argues, is to develop our skills in seeing the same situation in different ways. We can still take a pragmatic view, for example, in evidence-based medicine that we have a duty to use the best evidence available, but to be aware of the limitations of doing so, as what we are using is the process of interpretation and there may be other interpretations.

Methods for encouraging creative decision alternatives have been developed and tested. One is 'brainstorming', first proposed 60 years ago, where an unstructured group works together to develop a list of alternative solutions to a decision problem. The rules of brainstorming are:

- ideas should be freely expressed without considering their quality
- there is encouragement to modify and combine the ideas expressed
- there is no evaluation of the ideas until all have been stated.

Research into the value of this technique has shown mixed results compared with a number of individuals working on their own and then pooling their ideas, which is the approach used in the Delphi technique. Another technique, which may be worth trying if there is no one who already plays that role, is that of 'devil's advocate', where someone deliberately presents an opposite view to any consensus.

Summary

Difficulties with using and obtaining information effectively are as follows.

- Not thinking enough about:
  - what information is needed
  - the quality of the information
  - how quickly it can be obtained and whether that is soon enough.
- Not providing a challenge to individual/group myopia, which can lead to making a judgement too quickly, including rejecting unpalatable information.
- Reinventing the wheel because of lack of interest in learning from others.
- Too little impetus to take action on information collected.
- Human limitations in reasoning.

Knowledge is a broader term than information. It is now used in two senses: one, for the knowledge about a subject; two, for the new specialty of knowledge management which seeks to use and record the knowledge in people's heads.

There is a time-lag in the acceptance of new knowledge and an inertia that can prevent knowledge being used.

Knowledge is a result of interpretation: different people interpret evidence differently and time may give new perspectives.

How to improve

- Make a point of asking, and encouraging other members of the group to ask: 'What is the evidence for that?', including challenging what is being accepted as a fact.
- Make use of any colleague or member of a working group who is good at challenging accepted views.
- Seek to learn from the experience of others and, when appropriate, ask first what other people are doing about a problem that you are tackling. Intranet data bases can make this easier to do within the same organisation.
- Review what is being done to facilitate knowledge sharing.
- Find out which websites are of most use to you and use them.
- Consider what you know that your staff need to know, including what you have just learnt. Similarly what do you know that your boss does not and should know?
- Remember the common human errors in reasoning and take steps to guard against them.
- Check on the knowing–doing gap: what decisions have not been implemented and what consultancy and inspection reports have been neglected or only partially used?

References

1 McCall Jr MW, Kaplan RE (1985) *Whatever It Takes: decision makers at work*. Penguin, Harmondsworth, p. 14.
2 Nisbett R, Ross L (1980) *Human Inference: strategies and shortcomings of social judgment*. Prentice-Hall, New Jersey, pp. 292–3.
3 Bridges W (1990) *Surviving Corporate Transitions*. William Bridges and Associates.
4 Kotter J (1982) *The General Managers*. Harvard Business School, Boston, MA.

5 Peters TJ, Waterman Jr RH (1982) *In Search of Excellence: lessons from America's best-run companies*. Harper & Row, New York.

6 Drucker P (1999) *Management Challenges for the 21st Century*. Butterworth-Heinemann, Oxford.

7 Institute of Health Sciences (1999) *International Knowledge Partnership Health and Environment: promoting evidence-based decision making*. Institute of Health Sciences, Oxford, p. 2.

8 Antman EM, Lau J, Kupelnick B, Chalmers TC (1992) A comparison of results of meta-analyses of randomised control trials and recommendations of clinical experts. *JAMA*. **268**: 240–8; Ketley D and Woods KL (1993) Impact of clinical trials on clinical practice: example of thrombolysis for acute myocardial infarction. *Lancet*. **342**: 891–4.

9 Quoted in Richard Horton's review of Michael Bliss's *William Osler: a life in medicine* (2000) *New York Review of Books*. **xlvii**(9): 38.

10 Nutley S, Davies H (2000) Making a reality of evidence-based practice: some lessons from the diffusion of innovations. *Public Money and Mgmt*. **20**(4): 35–42.

11 *ibid*, p. 41.

12 Pfeffer J, Sutton RI (2000) *The Knowing–Doing Gap: how smart companies turn knowledge into action*. Harvard College, Boston, MA.

13 Stewart T (1997) *Intellectual Capital: the new wealth of organizations*. Nicholas Brealey, London.

14 Sauer C, Yetton P (1997) The right stuff: an introduction to new thinking about IT management. In: C Sauer, P Yetton and Associates (eds) *Steps to the Future: fresh thinking on the management of IT-based organisational transformation*. Jossey-Bass, San Francisco, CA.

15 Morgan G (1993) *Imaginisation: the art of creative management*. Sage, Beverly Hills, CA.

4

Are we doing a good job?

What evidence will we use to measure success and over what period of time?[1]

This should be a prime question for managers. Evidence-based managers will seek to answer it by improving the evidence base for assessing their performance. To do this requires deciding:

1 what is good performance
2 how good or bad is our performance
3 how to monitor what is happening
4 how to ensure that the monitoring is effective.

Evidence-based managers will be thoughtful and wide-ranging in seeking to answer the first question. They will search for the most reliable evidence to answer the other three and be alert to the ways in which the figures may be misleading.

What is good performance?

The answers will be determined by the context: in public companies, this will usually include how competitors are doing and what the market is expecting, and in the public sector, the criteria set by the government and the reactions of the public served. They will also be shaped by the values of the organisation, for example the importance given to customer and employee satisfaction.

Even within similar contexts, managers will differ in how broadly and critically they think about their performance. Some managers will seek only to meet the targets set from the top, others will be more probing in deciding how they should judge their performance. A simple illustration of such thinking comes from a GP* practice. All GPs should want to give a good service, but how they seek to judge whether they do, and hence what questions they ask themselves and what information they collect, differs. Some, for example, are more active than others in trying to find out about their patient population so as to judge what services need to be offered. They can also differ in how hard they try to assess their service and in the methods they use to do so.

Cookham Medical Centre provides a good example of an analysis of their patient population. The results of the analysis are obviously very different from that of a practice with a multi-ethnic and/or a very deprived population, which makes a similar analysis.

A different kind of question that GP practices can usefully ask about serving their patients is: When do they need the service? A simple analysis of patients' requests for an appointment would be likely to show that demand is highest on Monday morning, yet this may not be taken into account in the provision of surgery time, which may be, and in some practices still is, evenly divided across the days of the week. Retailers have more incentive to ask the question about the pattern of customer demand because they want to stock up

---

*General practitioner, the primary care doctor in Britain.

Box 4.1: Cookham Medical Centre

This case is included because it shows how a primary care practice can build up a good evidence base of the characteristics of their patient population and of their particular needs. This evidence can be used in deciding what is good performance, in addition to the targets set by government, and the knowledge of the patients' social situation can be used to try to improve attendance at regular clinics.

Cookham Medical Centre, a four-partner practice, was a 2000/2001 Beacon for the production of an annual report focusing on team development and clinical review. The annual report was chosen as an example of best practice in clinical governance. The practice also produces an annual clinical report which records clinical information and compares it with the previous year, including performance in the seven areas in which standards and service models have been set for Berkshire (the county where the practice is based). The annual report for 1999 shows the standard set, the achievements of the practice in that year and what should be done in 2000. It also compares their regular patients in December 1999 with the figures for the population in the UK in 1988, which was the latest census date. They have 50% fewer than the national average of 17–25-year-olds; the explanation they give is that in this mainly well-to-do area many are at university or need to live in a cheaper area. They have 100% more patients over 85 than the national average. The change in their practice population is 7 to 9% a year, so they say they find it easy to plan continuity of care, unlike one of their Beacon visitors, who had an annual 50% change of registration.

Both the annual report and the clinical report are well written and clearly presented. The annual report is wide ranging, with sections from all members of the team. One of the many interesting examples they give is of how they achieve a full attendance in their diabetic clinic, 96% over the years. This achievement is attributed to being flexible about times of appointment in consideration of patients' individual travel problems, work commitments and family problems. An interesting addition for readers of a later annual report is a 'Shipman'* audit in 2001, which gives the place of death, the cause and the doctor involved.

----

*Dr Shipman was the general practitioner convicted of killing many of his elderly patients.

and provide the staff to ensure that they can maximise sales. The Labour government's target, introduced in 2000, for how quickly patients should get an appointment to see the GP provided a spur to examining the appointment schedule and to considering what changes should be made to meet the target. The author's hope is that managers will not need an incentive, such as maximising sales, or an external pressure like meeting government targets, to want to ask searching questions about the service that is being provided.

Another example of trying to find out more about your patient population to see whether the service should be improved comes from the Southern Birmingham Community Health NHS Trust, now merged into the Birmingham Specialist Community Health NHS Trust, whose clinical audit department did an audit in 1997/98 to suggest how health/ social services provisions for older Yemeni people and their informal carers could be improved. One of the findings was that the assumption that older Yemeni people were being looked after by their families or relatives was a myth. Most lived in overcrowded bedsits in appalling living conditions. Another finding was that carers did not know that support for them is available. One of the actions taken as a result of the audit was the employment of Arabic-speaking staff across all agencies so that health knowledge and information could be provided in Arabic.

A good way of finding out what is good performance is to compare your own organisation with others.

How good or bad is our performance?

That question can only be answered satisfactorily if there are good comparative data. The NHS has lagged behind many other organisations in developing a good evidence base for judging performance. Alain Enthoven, the Stanford professor who has analysed the NHS over the years, deplored in a review published in 2000 that:

> *Even now, reliable quality-related information is virtually non-existent in the NHS. Many people appear afraid of it.... The importance of good information on quality and cost is not limited to market models. It is essential to any properly managed system, but especially to a centralised system. Without it, the center would have no way of recognising an improvement if one were to happen.*[2]

A research study in this country provided more specific evidence of the shortage of information for evaluating service performance. It was a study in England on the relationship between R&D and clinical practice in primary and secondary care, looking at cases of adult asthma and glue ear in children.[3] The researchers had chosen these two conditions for their ordinariness and had expected to include as part of their research data the process or outcome measures about these two. Yet they could not do so because they found nothing systematic, even for these ordinary conditions, for any of their sites, which included two teaching hospitals. Nor were they able to collect any systematic data on clinical behaviour. The analysis was, therefore, restricted to subjective data collected from physicians.

Readers may not be able to do anything about national inadequacies of information but, if they value evidence and recognise its importance in decision making, they can seek to improve the evidence that is available in their own organisation. A good example of this is given later in the chapter, in an audit of medical records.

Under Labour's NHS Plan 2000 there is a determined drive to develop performance data. There are detailed performance targets for many aspects of the health service from mental health to human resource management. Similarly, performance targets are being developed in other parts of the public sector. But it is too early to know, and we may never know, how reliable the performance data are and hence whether they will meet Enthoven's criticism of the lack of reliable data on quality-related information. Some performance targets can be measured much more reliably than others: the percentage of students getting A levels and their grades can be a much more accurate measure than the waiting time for appointments in hospitals, as the figures for that can be massaged.

The Good Hospital Guide, published in *The Sunday Times* in January 2001, reporting the results of the most comprehensive and authoritative measures of health service performance in Britain and Ireland, will help to ensure that managers and clinicians do know how their performance compares. However, the will to improve performance still needs to be there.

One method for assessing the organisation's performance is the balanced scorecard. This was introduced by Kaplan and Norton in the *Harvard Business Review* in 1992,[4] and developed in an article in 1996,[5] primarily as a tool for business, but it can be used in the public sector too; an example comes from the Tampere University Hospital and Pirkanmaa Hospital District in Finland (*see* Box 4.2). The balanced scorecard is a way of taking an overall view of what needs to be done to make the organisation efficient and effective. Central to the idea is that successful change needs to be integrated, hence the classic four scorecard areas are: financial, customer, internal processes, and learning and growth. A balanced scorecard approach is also to be used in Wales, according to the 2001 *Improving Health in Wales: a plan for the NHS and its partners*, to 'ensure certain targets are not achieved at the expense of others'.

Box 4.2: Target setting and monitoring in a Finnish university hospital and hospital district using a balanced scorecard

This case is included for the following reasons.
- A balanced scorecard is an integrated way of setting targets and measuring progress which was developed for, and used in, business but is suitable for any kind of organisation. It is a way of encouraging a good evidence base for decisions.
- It illustrates its use in a large Finnish university hospital and hospital district.

Tampere University Hospital is part of the Pirkanmaa Hospital District, which has a population of 440 000 and three smaller regional hospitals. Tampere University Hospital had 1377 beds in 1999 and, at the end of 1998, a staff of 3771. It provides specialised medical care for over a million Finns. The university hospital is also part of Finn-Medi, which is an international pool of medical research and healthcare technology of 12 000 people.

The balanced scorecard for Tampere University Hospital sets out the success factors and the targets in 2000. The success factors are given for:
- client view (customers in Kaplan and Norton)
- process view (internal processes in Kaplan and Norton)
- staff view (not included in Kaplan and Norton)
- improving activities (learning and growth in Kaplan and Norton)
- economy (financial in Kaplan and Norton).

Each of these is analysed under:
- success factors
- measurement tool
- attainable level
- follow-up frequency
- aims for long term, 3–5 years.

Among the measurements for client view are: hospital infections, e.g. for postoperative infections 8–10% is given as the attainable level; and scores on the patient satisfaction questionnaire, e.g. the attainable level for client assessment of visits to the outpatient department is better than 9.1 on a scale 4–10.

Among the success factors for process view is: activities of specialised medical and primary care are seamless, which is to be measured by the number of revisits, the time taken to send in medical reports and referral delay.

Among the long-term aims for process view is: 'action (including care programmes) is based on evidence-based knowledge and on the unified care management'.

Staff views are measured by a working climate measurement tool. Specific targets are given for the attainable level for key questions.

For many of the headings the measurement tool is given, but for some a new measurement tool will be developed in 2000, for example for the extent to which recommendations of good clinical practice are applied.

One of the measurements for the economic performance of the hospital district is that in the national benchmarking project it will be one of the three most economic hospital districts.

A study found that successful companies are increasingly using broad scorecards to monitor change and to widen the regular board review of the past year to include measures of behaviour and capability, as well as the more traditional ones of finance and market share.[6]

Another method for assessing the organisation's performance, which is also used in the public and private sectors, is benchmarking. This compares one organisation with others that are similar, or at least similar in the aspects being compared. Benchmarking can be used for comparison between similar processes in different organisations or between different parts of the same organisation. The process of benchmarking is divided into four stages: planning, analysis, communication of the findings and action; the analysis is to establish the gap between top benchmarks and own performance.

The first book on the subject was published in 1989,[7] although articles about it had been written earlier. A study in

1994 of the use of benchmarking in 1000 UK companies concluded that 78% used it and had found it to be helpful.[8] The main benefits found were:

- help in setting meaningful and realistic targets
- improvements in productivity
- gaining of insights into new or different approaches
- motivating employees by showing what was achievable.

The main problems reported were:

- difficulty in getting access to confidential information, especially about competitors, so that reason for restricting the exchange of information would not be a problem in the public sector
- lack of resources
- establishing the comparability of data from different organisations.

Despite the problems, most of the companies said they would expand their benchmarking work in the next five years.

One of the benefits described in the study, motivating employees by showing what is achievable, was strongly illustrated in an earlier study. This study, coordinated by the Massachusetts Institute of Technology (MIT), compared the performance of car assembly plants around the world, from 1985 to 1990, to identify the reasons for the differences.[9] The results of this comparison were so shocking that it was a trigger for the changes made in Western plants to emulate the achievements of the Japanese plants.

A case study cited in an article discussing benchmarking in the service industries,[10] is Yellow Pages, a division of British Telecommunications (BT), with 10 years' experience of benchmarking and 42 benchmarking projects. Crucial benchmarking projects are decided by the board of directors, and managers are encouraged to start their own. There is a 12-

step process for benchmarking, which includes: the importance attached to selecting benchmark partners, visiting, identifying practical solutions, planning action, implementing, keeping in touch and continuously improving. Financial, non-financial and operational performance measures are used with both qualitative and quantitative measures.

A criticism of benchmarking is that the data produced are partial and may overlook differences of context, for example in comparisons between Japanese and Western car manufacturers.

How to monitor what is happening

There are two aspects to this: first, to pick up what is happening and second, to understand it:

*The central problem of management in all its aspects ...
is to understand better the meaning of variation, and to
extract the information contained in variation.*
Dr Lloyd S Nelson, director of statistical methods for the Nashua Corporation, quoted by WE Deming[11]

Any large organisation has formal systems for identifying problems by showing when figures depart from expectations. These can be helpful, although, as any manager will know, they often raise problems about how reliable the figures are and whether they show a problem requiring action or are only a brief blip. Public health doctors face this kind of problem when there are reports of a few cases of a serious disease: are they isolated cases? the start of a trend? or of an epidemic? British public health doctors still do not know whether there will be few or very many further victims of the Creutzfeldt-Jakob disease. Similarly, a retail chain may not know whether a drop in sales is temporary or a sign of a drop in competitiveness, although comparisons with immediate competitors are a good indication.

Evidence-based managers will be alert to the importance of monitoring performance and proactive in thinking about what needs monitoring and in considering what methods to use to do so. They will do both regular monitoring and special monitoring of particular activities. Much of the regular monitoring may be specified for them by top management or, in the public sector, by the government. But there will still be scope for considering what other regular monitoring should be done to meet their particular circumstances and their own judgements of what is good performance. They should also be thinking about what activities may need a special check to identify likely weaknesses and to set standards for improvement. One example of a special check comes from the Birmingham Specialist Community Health NHS Trust.

Box 4.3: Birmingham Specialist Community Health NHS Trust trust-wide clinical records audit

This case is included because it is an audit of what is likely to be a common, but too often unexamined, problem of the state of clinical record keeping. The audit showed how much needed to be done to reach a good standard of record keeping and, after making recommendations for improvement, arranged for a re-audit.

A Clinical Records Working Party commissioned a pilot study (1997/98) that highlighted several areas of concern. It also drew on the evidence from a variety of reports, including reports from the Audit Commission, the Royal College of Surgeons and the standards for records and guidelines for record keeping previously adopted by one of the merged trusts. A wider audit was then undertaken in the trust so that the final report would carry greater authority.

Methodology
An appropriate sample-size activity was based on the activity of each division and a modified version of the pilot tool was developed in Formic. The data in each area were collected by small, trained, multi-professional project teams.

Results
These showed, as expected, that problems of legibility, signatures and mistakes were common in most areas of the trust. The overall standard of legibility across divisions varied from 58.5 to 95%. The number of records without any abbreviations varied between 1 and 36%. Twenty two percent of the records had mistakes, with only 2% amended according to the guidelines. Identification of clinicians at a later date is important, but in only 13% of the records was this possible.

Recommendations
- In areas of shared records, a common abbreviation list approved by the professions is to be developed and used to monitor variances.
- The importance of a clear, legible clinical record is to be stressed at all levels and regular reviews of records at divisional level should be considered.
- The importance of the entries being signed should be emphasised and staff made aware of a regularly monitored signature list. All new staff are to be informed of its existence at induction.
- Any entry in the record should be capable of being traced to a named individual and this should be stressed at induction sessions.
- The low level of compliance with the guidelines on mistakes shows there is a training issue for the divisions.

Each area of the trust is looking at the issues that require changes. The Clinical Records Steering Group is overseeing the implementation of recommendations. Action plans were developed and among the improvements made were staff training and development of agreed abbreviation lists for each speciality. Regular monitoring of clinical records is envisaged.

Another good example of a special check to see what is happening comes from the Cambridgeshire Health Authority, where research showed that the variations in peak demand in three acute hospitals were predictable. A study over three years showed similar peaks in demand each year in May/June, September/October and December/February. In the holiday period the daily activity was also predictable, particularly for Christmas and New Year.[12] This information is being used to improve planning for peak periods.

A thorough review of what is being monitored could usefully be made for each of the main activities of the organisation. This should look at what is not being monitored that should be. In human resource management, for example, a wide range of different forms of measurement can be made. Some organisations, particularly some US companies, conduct annual surveys to monitor employees' attitudes to their jobs and use the results as part of the assessment of a manager's performance. One measurement made in many organisations, particularly when they have staffing problems, is of labour turnover. This may be too broad a measure to be useful; often more detailed measurement may be necessary, for example: who is leaving? (this question may be broken down by occupation, sex and age); how long have they been in the job?; why are they leaving?

One common measure of the quality of the service is complaints. In hospitals, one measurement that is often cited is the number of complaints and whether this has changed; sometimes also the number of letters of praise. But as in most measures of performance, it is important to examine the assumptions that are being made about the measure. For example, is it meaningful to make a straight comparison with number of complaints over time? Should we take account of what other factors may have influenced people's willingness to complain? Are complaints a good measure of the level of satisfaction? Perhaps some, even many, people do not complain even though they are dissatisfied? Measuring the

number of complaints is a reactive measure of patient satisfaction, a more proactive one is to ask patients specific questions about their experience. Again there is a choice about
when this is done, which may affect the response. In the
assessment of management training programmes, for
example, it has been found that participants give a different
evaluation at the end of the programme from that at a later
date.

Despite the government drive for more attention to the
users in the public sector, it is the private sector that can
provide many of the best examples of checking on customer
satisfaction. The motivation in a private company is different,
it is to ensure a satisfied customer who will buy again and
recommend their product. In a public service where the
demand exceeds the resources, the motivation is obviously
different, but useful lessons can still be learnt by studying
what is done by the better firms with which you deal.

How to ensure that the monitoring is reliable

Evidence-based managers will actively explore the reliability
of their monitoring. Good questions to ask of any monitoring
system are:

- What is it providing evidence of?
- Are there incentives for distorting the information?
- In what ways may the information provided be mis-
leading?
- Is the information sufficiently up to date to be useful?
- Is it accurate? If not, what are the likely sources of inaccu-
racy?
- Is the monitoring actually taking place?

Budgets are a good example of the uses and abuses of monitoring systems. They are a useful planning tool and, as such,

encourage staff to pay attention to future financial needs and to the relative financial priorities within the monies available. They can also help to monitor whether current expenditure is in line with the budget, so that divergences can be identified. However, any reader is likely to know of their limitations as a control tool. It is common to ask for more than you need because you expect the budget to be cut or because it would be nice to have some extra money. Where you cannot keep surplus on the budget at the end of the year, there is the rush to find a project to spend it on. If one expenditure heading is likely to be more favourably viewed than another, there may be attempts to stretch the interpretation of what can be included under that heading. These are just three familiar examples of how monitoring systems often do not work as they are intended to.

The last question in the list above may be surprising to some readers. It comes from the author's experience in her first research study in the NHS back in the mid-1960s. It was a study of the response to a 1964 Ministry circular requiring action on monitoring time spent waiting for an outpatients appointment and time spent waiting in the outpatients department – some ministerial concerns have a long history! The performance standards for both were set out in the circular: the waiting time for an appointment should not exceed two weeks and for waiting time in the outpatients department, 75% of patients should be seen within half an hour of their appointment time, with not more than 3% waiting an hour. The research sought to find out reactions in the NHS to the circular. Nearly all those interviewed said they kept both kinds of waiting 'continuously under review', which was used ironically as the title for the research report,[13] because when questioned further, one-third had made no attempt in the past five years to check the working of their appointment system and very few of the others reviewed it regularly.

Monitoring systems may cease to serve a useful function

and some may never have done so because those who supply the information do not believe in the utility of the system or are afraid to give accurate information. All systems for monitoring what is happening need to be looked at critically: first when they are going to be introduced, to ask what can go wrong and why? Later they need to be reviewed to see whether they are really serving the purpose intended.

So far the questions posed have been about existing monitoring systems or, at least, about what managers think is being monitored. Just as, perhaps even more, important is what is not being monitored. Organisations, even similar organisations, can differ widely in how much and what kind of monitoring they do and hence in their evidence base for decisions.

Avoiding bad surprises

There are bound to be unexpected problems, hence trouble-shooting is one aspect of managers' jobs. In politics, as Macmillan said, the main problem is 'events', that is, the unexpected problems that arise, like foot and mouth disease in Britain in 2001. Even though there will always be unexpected problems, the number can be cut down by good monitoring. The importance of monitoring is shown in spectacular failings, such as not identifying much sooner that Dr Shipman was a dangerous GP and thus allowing him to murder many patients over the years, or not following up on reports of a faulty rail at Hatfield, which could have prevented a fatal rail crash there later. The importance of good monitoring is greatest in organisations where poor monitoring can result in injury or death, such as dangerous plants, air, rail and hospitals, hence the particular importance of risk management in such organisations. In Chapter 6, there is a description of how British Airways monitors deviations from flight norms in order to learn how to improve safety.

There is no close parallel with the kind of monitoring in organisations using a different technology, but avoiding bad surprises as far as possible should still be a major aim.

It may be wise to review the monitoring systems that exist to ask whether they do provide a good early warning system. A good student project – which would cost little or no money – would be to do a check over the past couple of years to see what problems have been identified and whether there are others that have arisen that should have been identified but were not.

One of the things that goes wrong with problem identification is that warnings are ignored. Military historians have reported glaring examples that led to unnecessary loss of life. Such failures can come from being too set on your own interpretation or because of poor communication between different specialist divisions. There seems no reason to think that the armed services are uniquely prone to such failures, rather that it is the seriousness of their crucial decisions that has encouraged historians to trace what happened.[14]

In the health services, over the years there has been an awareness of the need to monitor and reduce the incidence of adverse incidents. Yet in the NHS far too little has been done. Most recently a report by an expert group on the subject, *An Organisation with a Memory*,[15] chaired by Liam Donaldson, the Chief Medical Officer, said:

> *Guidance on the reporting of adverse incidents in the NHS stretches back over 40 years, but there is still no standardised reporting system, nor indeed a standard definition of what should be reported.*[15]

A study in 1999[16] found that NHS trusts, in default of any national system, varied considerably in what they did about this, in whether they had reporting systems covering the whole organisation and in whether they provided guidance about what to report. In response to the inadequacies shown in *An Organisation with a Memory*, a National Patient Safety Agency was established in 2001 to gather details of adverse incidents in NHS hospitals across Britain.

Summary

Evidence-based managers should be asking themselves four questions. First, what is good performance for the work of my unit? They should not try just to meet the targets set from above, but also seek to really understand the work of their unit and to ask searching question about how good performance should be judged. An example is given of questions that GPs can ask themselves. Second, how does our performance compare with others: are we good or bad? Evidence-based managers should think broadly and critically in answering this question. The contribution that two techniques, the balanced scorecard and benchmarking, can make to tackling this question is described and illustrated. Third, how can we best monitor what is happening? Regular monitoring is important and so is being alert to what is not being, and should be, monitored. An example is given of an audit of how well clinical records were being kept. Fourth, how to ensure that monitoring yields accurate and timely information. There is a need to avoid bad surprises and to reduce their incidence by better monitoring which does give good warnings of problems.

How to improve

- What is the best example in your organisation of how well you tackle each of the four questions? What can you learn from that, that you can use elsewhere?
- How broadly and critically have you thought about what is good performance? Where should you start doing so?

- Where else should you be seeking to improve performance outside the targets you have been set?
- Are you using benchmarking? If not, find an organisation that is comparable to yours to do so. It could also be useful to try and make some comparisons with organisations that are in a different sector from yours.
- Seek to interest an MBA student in developing a balanced scorecard for your organisation.
- What are you not monitoring that needs to be monitored?
- Are you getting adequate warning of problems? If not, what can be done to get a better warning system going?
- When and where have checks been made of the reliability of the monitoring information? Where should checks be made?
- Build organisational memory by embedding the knowledge from reviews of performance into databases and work processes.

References

1 Homa P (1998) What's your evidence? *Health Management*, **July**: 19. This is one of the questions suggested for an evidence-based approach.
2 Enthoven AC (2000) In pursuit of an improving National Health Service. *Health Affairs*. **19**: 3, 107.
3 Dopson S, Dawson S, Miller R, Sutherland R (1999) Getting research into practice: the case of glue ear. *Quality in Healthcare*. **8**: 108–18.
4 Kaplan R, Norton D (1992) The balanced scorecard – measures that drive performance. *Harvard Business Review*. **Jan–Feb**: 71–7.
5 Kaplan R, Norton D (1996) Using the balanced scorecard as a strategic management system. *Harvard Business Review*. **Jan–Feb**: 75–85.
6 Ruddle K, Feeny D (1997) *Transforming the Organisa-*

tion: new approaches to management measurement and leadership. Templeton Executive Briefing, Templeton College, Oxford.

7 Camp RC (1989) *Benchmarking: the search for industry best practices that lead to superior performance.* ASQC Quality Press, Milwaukee, WI.

8 Coopers & Lybrand/CBI (1994) *Survey of Benchmarking in the UK.* CBI, London.

9 Womack J, Jones D, Roos D (1990) *The Machine that Changed the World.* Rawson Macmillan, New York.

10 Simpson M, Kondouli D (2000) A practical approach to benchmarking in three service industries. *Total Quality Management.* **11**: 4–6, S623–630.

11 Deming WE (1982, 1986) *Out of the Crisis: quality, productivity and competitive position.* Cambridge University Press, Cambridge, p. 20.

12 Jewell T, Spiers H (2000) Tales of the expected. *Health Service Journal.* **2 Nov**: 30–1.

13 Stewart R, Sleeman J (1967) *Continuously Under Review: a study of the management of out-patient departments.* Occasional Papers on Social Administration No. 20. G Bell & Sons, London.

14 Dixon J (1976) *On the Psychology of Military Incompetence.* Jonathan Cape, London.

15 Department of Health (2000) *An Organisation with a Memory: report of an expert group on learning from adverse events in the NHS.* The Stationery Office, London.

16 Dineen M, Walsh K (1999) Incident reporting in the NHS. *Health Care Risk Report.* **March**.

5

Improving decision making

A muddled mind creates muddles around it. Management is largely a question of decision, and decisions cannot be properly taken unless the mind is clear about objectives and priorities.[1]

...the decision-making process will seldom go unaffected by the swirl of managerial demands.[2]

Decision making is a central aspect of management. There is only limited value in improving the management of information if the decision-making process is poor, so anyone who wants to practise evidence-based management should review the effectiveness of decision making in their organisation. Fortunately, decision making has attracted a great deal of research over the years so there is good evidence to draw on when discussing ways of improving it.[3]

The evidence-based manager will realise the importance of trying to ensure that decision making is based on as good evidence as can sensibly be obtained within the time and cost constraints. It is obviously worth making more effort to do so for important decisions than for lesser ones. So concern for the evidence base for decisions is one characteristic of the evidence-based manager. Another is a desire to improve decision making and an interest in learning how to do so.

One of the findings of a number of research studies is that decision making is a process that goes through different stages and there are lessons about potential weaknesses at each stage. Another is that decisions vary along a continuum from programmed to unprogrammed. The programmed decisions can be left to more junior staff because procedures and protocols for making them can be devised. It is the non-programmed decisions, which are the unfamiliar strategic ones, that provide the challenge to managers.

Stages in decision making

For a decision-making process to start you have to be aware of the need to make a decision, although some decisions take place without conscious thought, as anyone can check for themselves. It is fortunate that that happens because it saves time and effort. Conscious decision making may stem from the recognition of a problem, a deviation from what is considered desirable or from a desire to make an improvement.

One way of analysing the effectiveness of decision making is to think of it as a logical process that passes through the following stages:

- recognition of a problem or an opportunity
- defining the problem
- identifying what information is required
- collecting the information
- reviewing the information collected
- identifying possible solutions and examining their pros and cons
- selecting one
- implementation.

This is a sequence, but it may be necessary to cycle back at any stage and it is often wise to start the preparation for implementation in the early stages so that key people become convinced of the need for change. Evidence-based management is relevant at each stage of the decision process because mistakes can be made at any stage. Box 5.1 summarises what can go wrong.

Box 5.1:   What can go wrong in decision making

- Identifying the wrong problem or opportunity
- Problems in information used (see Figures 3.1 and 3.2)
- Not persuading others that a change is necessary
- Too narrow a search for possible solution
- Commitment to the solution too soon
- Poor choice of solution
- No or poor implementation planning
- No implementation

It is a mistake to attach too much importance to 'the decision'. Decision making is not a single event but a process that can only be called successful when the hoped-for improvement or change has been achieved. There may be a decision recorded in board minutes, but as one IT manager reported when the introduction of a new system had been approved, he was surprised when the chief executive's comment was 'good luck'. He had not realised that the board's agreement was only one step on the way. Another reason why the idea of 'the decision' can be unhelpful is that decisions, particularly about strategy, may emerge from a series of small steps rather than from a particular point in time.

There are logical steps in the decision process, but it is often necessary to go back to an earlier stage because of the amount of uncertainty, and even confusion, there can be in the more difficult decisions. This is well put by Burns, an early researcher in leadership:

> *Executive decision-making is not a series of single linear acts like baking a pie. It is a process, ... that stretches back into a murky past and forward into a murkier future. (It is) a turbulent stream ... a twisted, unshapely, halting flow.*[4]

Practitioners of evidence-based management cannot change this reality, but they can learn to avoid the pitfalls that exist at each stage. They can start by trying to improve their ability to identify and to prioritise problems. Many problems are messy and ill-defined, but even when a problem appears clear-cut, this can be deceptive. The manager may be told of a problem and of the solution to it. Both pieces of information may be wrong or misleading. Managers who want to practise evidence-based management have to be willing to live with the ambiguity and uncertainty that come from a thoughtful and searching approach to deciding what the problem and the most promising solution are. Otherwise they can be in danger of being like the hen in the experiment, with spectacles that altered its focus so that it was always pecking in the wrong place for the corn.

One of the reasons a problem may not get recognised correctly is that it bridges several specialties or departments. Specialisation is an organisational means of creating units with expertise in dealing with particular types of problem. This has obvious advantages, but the disadvantage is expressed in the phrase 'falling between two stools', so that a problem that crosses professional or departmental boundaries may not get recognised. This can be a particular problem in the public sector, where the current emphasis in the UK on 'joined-up thinking' still has a long way to go.

Sometimes the problem may be all too well known and then the problem becomes how to tackle it, or perhaps first how to summon the will to tackle it.

Tackling well-known problems

Examples in the NHS of such well-known, long-standing problems are: long waiting times; bed blocking particularly by elderly people living alone; and cancellation of elective surgery patients to deal with emergencies. It is easier to tackle such long-standing problems when there is an external impetus for doing so, because then they claim that scarce commodity, managerial attention. In companies, this is likely to come from top management, often in response to competitive pressures. In the public service the impetus is likely to come from ministers.

Boxes 5.2 and 5.3 show different approaches to tackling a long-standing problem, which had now become a government requirement; both were awarded a Beacon for their success in doing so. The case studies are written so as to emphasise the use of evidence in decision making, to point to what evidence there is, and its limitations, and, in the first case, to weaknesses in the decision-making process identified by a panel of judges.

Box 5.2: Pre-assessment and care management at Greenwich Healthcare NHS Trust

This case is included for the following reasons:
- it is an example of the successful tackling of a long-standing and common problem
- it identified the reason for bed blocking and devised a successful solution to it
- it is an example of successful collaboration between health and social services
- it also shows what further information would have improved its evidence base.

It was one of four projects within a wider project, Collaborative Pathways Project Team, all to do with improving the patient's journey through the system, maximising current resource allocation and ultimately reducing overall waiting times. Only this project is described here because it was the most successful of the four.

The pre-assessment and care management subgroup, like the other three, developed its own timetable within the overall time frame using GANNT charts, one of the most commonly used tools for scheduling events. It was developed by HL Gannt in 1917 and is one of the first recorded attempts to relate activity in time for purposes of scheduling.

The overall project was nominated for the NHS Team of the Year Award. They did not reach the finals but were highly commended for the quality of the work. The project planning was described as excellent, with good use of GANNT charts and meeting minutes. Resources were clearly identified on commencement of the project. An area suggested for improvement was that it was not clear how the GANTT charts were updated and used to track progress. This comment points to *the need not just to try to plan the schedule at the start against time but to continue to check whether the work is going to plan and if not, to plan the repercussions of a delay in any aspect.* This criticism is mainly relevant to the other, and more complex parts, of the overall project but is included here because it can be an easy mistake to make.

The pre-assessment and care management subgroup identified the problem of bed blocking as being due to: late referrals to social services and the inability to meet social care needs in a short time; and not giving patients advance information about provision for social care needs. The solution identified and adopted was to base two care managers within the pre-assessment clinic so that social needs can be identified. A similar system of referral of ortho-paedic patients to physiotherapists and occupational therapists was also introduced.

This early identification of social needs meant that care managers had more time to plan for the necessary care, and discussing aftercare with the patient and their relatives before admission enabled many to make their own preparations for it, having had time to consider the options. This appears to reduce the need for and level of care packages. 'Appears' because it is based on the experience of the hospital care manager, Neil Jones, rather than on measurement. In his experience, previously about

80% of referrals to care management ended up with a care package, whereas now that patients can discuss their care needs and plan for them before admission only about 25% need care packages.

The decrease from 11.1 days to 8.6 days in the average length of stay of patients referred to care management from the outset of the project in May 1998 to December 1999 is attributed to these changes. However, the extent to which the reduction in the average length of stay can be attributed to the pre-assessment of social care needs is not known. It can be argued that it is the reduction that matters most rather than the reason for it, but in evidence-based management it is better to know, as far as possible, what causes changes. Similarly it would be useful to have firmer information about the apparent reduction in the need for care packages.

The achievements of the whole project were recognised by being made a Beacon in the first year of the scheme.

The second example of tackling a long-standing problem, that of waiting lists, was not part of a larger project, but comes from the orthopaedic department in the University Hospital Aintree. It was an initiative of the physiotherapists and required an acceptance of a change in their role.

Box 5.3: Agreed use of physiotherapists to reduce orthopaedic waiting list at University Hospital Aintree

The case is included because it is an example of careful planning of a novel change in clinical practice using evidence and a step-by-step introduction as a means of gaining acceptance.

Origins of the scheme
There was a clear need for action to reduce the orthopaedic waiting list, which was in excess of 5000, with some patients waiting over two years – much longer than the norm for the government initiative to reduce waiting lists. Hence suggestions for

ways of doing this were likely to be welcomed, provided they were considered acceptable by the consultants and GPs concerned and the patient.

The only documented evidence of changes in the roles of physiotherapists and consultants is an article that had not been published at the start of the scheme and was not known until later.[5]

Aim
To reduce the outpatient waiting list by introducing physiotherapy-led orthopaedic clinics for those patients whose referral suggests that physiotherapy assessment and treatment is the most appropriate initial intervention.

Steps in achieving the aim
A search through the waiting lists by specialist physiotherapists showed that many patients could be managed by specialist physiotherapists.
- Agreed with orthopaedic consultants, first two then six, that their waiting lists can be reviewed by physiotherapists to agreed criteria to see which patients can be assessed and treated by specialist physiotherapists.
- Acquired funding through the waiting list initiative.
- Started the selection on 21 May 1998.
- Consultants validated the selection of the first 100 patients and then left it to the physiotherapists.

The referring GP receives a letter saying that their referral has been reviewed by an orthopaedic consultant and that it is deemed more appropriate for their patient to be assessed first by a specialist musculoskeletal physiotherapist. GPs are asked to reply within a set time if they are not happy with this. If they are not, the patient, instead of receiving a faster appointment with the physiotherapist, returns to their same position on the consultant's waiting list. A full report of the outcome is sent to the referring GP.

Patients were also offered a choice of accepting the appointment with the specialist physiotherapist or remaining on the waiting list in the same position as before.

Later the process was changed with the agreement of the local primary care groups (the first stage of further changes in the devolution of commissioning to GPs) so that patients selected for appointments with specialist physiotherapists were immediately given an appointment without first gaining GP approval or patient permission.

The change had various staffing implications which had to be tackled. For the initial pilot, existing staff were seconded to manage the scheme as a suitably qualified person could not be recruited, given the shortages. Agency staff were employed to cover the normal workload. A full-time clerical officer was recruited. Permanent staff were recruited for subsequent years.

Extra pay was given for time spent assessing patients, as doing so extended the role of the physiotherapist.

As expected the change increased the physiotherapy waiting list. This was resolved in later years by funding an additional senior post.

Conditions considered necessary for success apart from funding
These are given by Arlene Allan, physiotherapy services manager, as:
- well-trained senior grade physiotherapists who have postgraduate training in the musculoskeletal specialty. The staff used have at least five years' postgraduate experience in the field
- good relationships between the consultants and the physiotherapists. They had worked together and the physiotherapists thus knew the criteria the surgeons followed when selecting patients for surgery
- adequate dedicated clerical support.

Outcomes and evaluation
The outcomes that would be audited were agreed as part of the scheme. Monitoring after three months using a specially designed database showed that the target of removing 400 patients from the orthopaedic waiting list had been achieved. Additional funding with a target of 1000 patients in the year was also achieved. At the end of the first year, out of 714 patients assessed, only 156 in the opinion of the physiotherapists required a consultant appointment, suggesting GPs were not making best use of their open access to physiotherapy.

The scheme is developing in a number of ways. There is now consolidated funding for 100 patients a year to be managed by the physiotherapists and extra non-recurring funding to clear an additional 1758 patients by July 2001.

The scheme became a Beacon and has been contacted and visited by many other departments with a view to developing similar schemes.

Lessons from studies of decision making

A large-scale study across different kinds of organisations provides a guide for improving major decision making: it reports how managers went about making such decisions and which tactics worked best. Readers who are interested only in a summary of management research should skip the next few paragraphs and start reading again at the emboldened paragraph on p. 105, beginning 'Overall, Nutt concludes ....'

Paul Nutt studied the tactics used for major decision making in different departments in medium to large organisations, in companies, the public sector and the not-for-profit sector in the US and Canada. He took as his main indicator of the success of decision making whether the decision was implemented. He followed 365 decisions in different departments for two years to see what changes there were during that time. The success of a decision was determined by whether it was still operational two years later and the degree to which it was. By this test half of them failed.[6] And there is no reason to think that a similar study carried out in the UK or in other countries would have been more encouraging about managers' success in major decision making. The study found that most of the failures were due to factors within the managers' control.

Nutt identified the most successful tactics used at three of the stages in major decision making. His research suggested a stage, 'direction setting', which is a useful addition to the customary analysis of stages, described earlier. He distinguished four tactics here and described their relative success.

The first, generating ideas, is the most common tactic and the least successful. The danger of this tactic is that coming up with an idea for a solution early on encourages managers to focus on a single solution. 'Commitment became a trap that often produced failure.' This can be made worse over time by concern for sunk costs, fears of admitting failure and a reluctance to abandon the project or to start over. The history of the Dome, as Britain's major millennium project, could be seen as one of the big public examples of this.

The second tactic is problem solving, which was often unsuccessful because too little attention was given to problem definition; this may happen because managers are too keen to find out what is wrong and to fix it quickly, rather than make an adequate exploration of the problem. Another reason it can be unsuccessful is that defining a problem can encourage defensiveness unless an effort is made to show why a change is needed (see the fourth tactic).

The third tactic, the second most commonly used, was objective setting, which had better results than the first two. Nutt suggests that although objective setting is known to be a good idea, it is seldom practised 'because managers have a bias towards action and fear of being seen as indecisive. Action-oriented managers see objectives as an academic exercise'. As one would expect, the chance of success improves when a realistic objective is set.

The fourth tactic, and the least often used, was the most successful. Nutt calls it 'intervening in the process', that is, showing the need for action. It is too easy for managers to assume that their concern for action to improve current performance is shared by others: decisions are more likely to be implemented successfully if managers spend time early on seeking to convince others that action is needed and accords with agreed goals.

Nutt also examined what tactics the managers used for identifying the options for decision taking. He distinguished between imposed solutions and discovery ones. In imposed solutions, the managers quickly decided what should be done. In only about a third of the decisions did they explore various options. The three tactics for discovering a solution were: adapting the ideas of others; an active search for possible solutions; and designing a solution themselves.

A relatively rare tactic in searching for a solution, but one with a good record of success, was to examine what several organisations were doing in this area and select the best features of each; similarly to examine different consultancy packages as a basis for producing a clearly defined tender brief. Those who did not do this risked being sold a system that did not fit their needs. Time pressure or limited access to what others are doing were two reasons for not making multiple comparisons more often. Limited access is likely to be less of a problem in the public than in the private sector. Very few of the organisations sought to design their own solution because doing so was seen as more risky than adopting that of others or using consultants. Nutt suggests that the motivations to be pragmatic are stronger than those to be innovative.

Nutt identified four tactics for implementation. The first, and most successful, he called 'intervention'; it was used by only 7% of the organisations. As he points out, 'managers often assume that the concern that motivated them to act is obvious to others', and that they agree about its importance. This assumption is often wrong, so that the most successful tactic was to start trying to persuade people that change is necessary early on. He gives as an example, what was done to gain support for introducing a burn care service in a hospital, which was to show how this could be funded and how it could help medical recruitment to have such a service.

The second, and well-known, tactic for facilitating implementation of a change is participation, such as creating task forces with key individuals as members. This was used in fewer than a fifth of the decisions, with managers saying that they knew of the value of participation but found it difficult, partly because of the time it takes and partly because of a feeling of loss of control. The researchers found no examples of comprehensive participation where all stakeholders are involved in finding concerns and suggesting solutions.

The third tactic for facilitating implementation is persuasion. This was used in 40% of the decisions studied but with a lower success rate than for intervention or participation. The main persuasion tactic was gathering expert documentation rather than dealing with the concerns of the key people affected by the decision and thus gaining their acceptance. The fourth tactic was just to announce a decision, explaining a new policy and when it will go into effect. Such edicts were made in 40% of the decisions and had the highest failure rate.

Overall, Nutt concludes from his research that managers can improve their chances of making successful decisions, that is ones where implementation stands the test of time. Managers must personally manage the decision-making process, championing the need for a change, taking time to explore the problem, identifying more than one option for solution and dealing with barriers to action by involving as many of the stakeholders as possible in the search for a solution and in planning for implementation. He says that his conclusions are supported by the results of 30 other studies.

Nutt has shown the need to improve decision making and so have other studies. A British group of researchers studied investment decisions and identified a tension between two different approaches: the computational, characterised by step-by-step planning and the calculation of an optimal solution, and inspirational decision making. They suggest that both are present and necessary in the iterative process of decision making, because at times inspiration – acting on hunches

– will be required when action has to be taken with incomplete information.[7]

Janis and Mann, in a study of how people behave when making decisions under stress, identified defensive avoidance as being one way of coping.[8] Defensive avoidance can be achieved by procrastination, buck passing and bolstering, that is, by magnifying the attractions of the chosen solution and decreasing those of the alternatives. Janis and Mann claimed that it is a common occurrence in the military, law enforcement agencies, hospitals and school systems. They were talking about US organisations, but there seems no reason to think that similar patterns of behaviour are not found in organisations in other countries.

Janis and Mann give some ways of preventing a group from indulging in defensive avoidance. The first two would be useful in any policy-planning group; the remainder are more time consuming so only appropriate for major policy decisions:

- when setting up a policy-planning group the chairman or chief executive should give a neutral briefing to encourage an atmosphere of open inquiry
- the group chairman should encourage members to air objections and doubts
- the group should sometimes divide into two, meeting separately with different chairmen, and then sort out their differences in the main group
- one or more qualified colleagues should be invited to different meetings and encouraged to challenge the group's view
- after reaching a preliminary consensus about what to do, there should be a second chance meeting where every member is expected to express their residual doubts, as vividly as possible, to encourage rethinking the whole issue before reaching a decision.[9]

The role of intuition in decision mak

We need to control the subjective bias inherent human, but not to lose the advantages of our in which is immediate insight without reasoning. So far has been a very analytical account of how to improve dec sion making: we can learn to make better decisions by improving our analysis. We should strive to do so and ways of doing this are summarised at the end of the chapter. But we also need to be aware of the reality of decision making: it is not, and cannot be, a wholly unemotional, analytical process. Obviously managers cannot do their jobs well on intuition alone, because it may not be working or it may be wrong, but it is a faculty that can and should be nurtured and used.

In one research study, 60 experienced professionals in the US were interviewed about their views on, and use of, intuitive decision making.[10] Over 90% said they used intuition together with data analysis for some decisions; some said they always used intuition, others less often and a few that they rarely used it. The professionals thought that intuition developed from their experience and learning.

In another study a dozen senior American business executives were interviewed and observed for 25 days to discover how they thought about problems.[11] The researcher found that the executives used intuition for five different purposes, to:

- sense when a problem exists
- carry out well-learned patterns of behaviour quickly and without thinking – the most common example would be driving a car
- synthesise isolated bits of information into an integrated picture
- check on a formal analysis to identify holes in the data
- come quickly to a solution for a familiar problem.

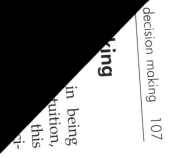

important part that experience
ın also be part of it: there may
ıptions being considered is not
ling or a sense that the facts put
at further inquiry is necessary.
spoke of a learned ability to

ɔy the American professionals
ınd again there is no reason to
.... will not be true of professionals and executives in
other countries – it is worth trying to make it work well for
you. Sometimes only the analytical approach is appropriate
to the problem, because the problem is clear and so are the
information and the most appropriate solution. All that is
needed then is good planning at all stages, including the
implementation, and the determination to follow through.
Mostly, analysis and intuition should be used together: the
type of problem faced will determine what mix of the two is
required.

Intuition may need nurturing, particularly by those who
have had a long analytical training. One well-known technique is working on a problem or a difficult report before it is
required so that your mind will go on working on it when
you are doing other things: some people call this 'instructing
their unconscious'. Another is making sure that you capture
ideas, in the hope that they are bright ideas. Notes about
such fringe thoughts, with the initials FT, is one way to do so.

There is a danger that emphasising evidence-based
management could create an organisational culture that
discourages the use of intuition. Yet a research-based
approach to decision making should mean that the value of
intuition, which has been shown by research, is recognised,
as well as the need for an evidence-based approach. Decision
making is often difficult and hard to get right so we should
use all the different methods we can, and cultivating intuition
is one of them. The times when intuition is most likely to

make a helpful contribution are:

- when decisions need to accord with the organisation's values, where an intuitive sense that what is proposed is not right can be helpful
- when a decision has to be made quickly
- when there are no policies, guidelines or expert guidance that are relevant
- when quantitative analyses require a check and an ability to question their limitations.

There are, however, dangers in relying too much on intuition. Managers can then be impatient with details, reach conclusions too quickly and ignore relevant facts. They may follow an inspiration which is mistaken. In problem solving analysis and intuition need to go together.

As the study cited above suggests, most managers combine the rational and the intuitive approaches, but some are much more strongly one way than the other, as anyone who has filled in the Myers Briggs selection test will know. Both approaches are necessary, so a manager who is much stronger in one direction than the other needs to be complemented by someone who is stronger in the opposite direction, which is a key lesson drawn about the differences shown by the Myers Briggs test. The rational manager is the one who will find the idea of evidence-based management most appealing, but unlike the intuitive manager will prefer to think of knowledge as objective. The suggestion that there are different ways of interpreting a situation can be very uncomfortable for those who like to see things as clear-cut. The intuitive manager is more likely to be able to do this, and to like doing so, but all can learn to recognise that there are different ways of seeing the same situation and that they should seek to do so. Psychologists have visual games which make the point by asking different people to define the subject of a drawing.

Politics in decision making

One of the lessons from research into decision making is that, at the top, it is concerned with the allocation and exercise of power in organisations. The issues, which are often not made explicit, are:

- who is involved in the making of decisions
- who is left out or kept out
- who can exercise influence on:
  - the composition of the decision-making group
  - what gets on the agenda and its order as that can influence the amount of attention given
  - the decision that is reached
  - whether, how and when it is implemented.

In public bureaucracies, these issues of power are more prescribed but they still exist.

The picture that emerges from some of the studies of actual decision making over time is of multiple, competing interest groups vying for supremacy when there are decisions being discussed that affect their interests. This gives a quite different explanation of what is going on than an account of decisions as the result of rational choice. It reflects, too, the difference between those who see organisations as cohesive, with their members having a unified view, and those who see them, more realistically, as pluralistic with many different viewpoints and interests.

A useful correction to those who believe that decision making is always a very political activity comes from a study by a team at Bradford University of 150 decisions in 30 organisations in the private and public sectors.[12] They found that this was true for about a third of the decisions, but that the others were more deliberative and less contentious. In a third of the decisions, the outcome was not in doubt, sometimes because there was only one realistic option but sometimes because of prior agreement among the key players. The process of decision making varied greatly depending on the type of problem, particularly whether it was one where different interests were affected by it. The researchers concluded that:

> *There is no top decision which does not call for the know-how to deal with the complexity of problems and the 'know-who' to deal with the politicality of interests.*[13]

Many decisions require balancing the interests of different stakeholders both within and outside the organisation: the amount of power that different groups of stakeholders can exercise will affect the decision process, including the actual decision and how implementation goes. These interests, and the political activity that often accompanies them, are based on values. Clashes of values are particularly common in non-profit organisations because members may feel very strongly about the values underlying the organisation but interpret them differently. For example, doctors will want to do the best for the individual patient, whereas managers have to take account of the needs of broad groups of patients and of the ability of the organisation to be financially viable.

Non-decisions

What a curious idea! Yet it is another of the findings of some researchers into decision making. Non-decisions are the issues that are not considered suitable for discussion so they are avoided, because they go against the interests of powerful individuals or groups, or because they do not accord with the organisational culture. This view of decision making suggests that you cannot discover all the major issues and problems by looking at what is being decided. Some of the future decisions may come from an event that makes it too difficult to continue to avoid the topic: doing something about poorly performing or negligent doctors is a recent example, which had to be tackled after several much-publicised examples of grossly negligent and even criminal doctors. This had been a non-decision for a long time because of the power of doctors and their belief that regulating doctors was a professional matter and should be controlled by the medical profession. What could be called another form of non-decision is where it is tacitly accepted that the decision has already been made, even though there may be a show of going through a discussion about making the decision.

Group decision making

The relative merits of individuals or groups in making effective decisions have also been studied. Defining the problem and choosing a solution are likely to be slower in a group, but implementation is quicker. Fortunately for managers in the public service, and especially in the health service, which has so many groups taking decisions, a review of research into decision making suggests that groups are preferable in the following circumstances:[14]

- when getting acceptance of the decision is likely to be difficult and essential for implementation
- when it is a complex decision requiring different expertise
- when creating ideas and remembering information are important
- when there needs to be a division of labour because no single person can comprehend it all.

Since many of these circumstances often apply in the health service the large amount of time that health service managers spend in meetings can be explained, but much could be done to improve the use of that time. Many of these improvements are well known, but not necessarily practised, like good chairing. One of the decisions that managers in many organisations, particularly in the NHS, need to make is how to improve the effectiveness and efficiency of meetings, which should also help to improve the satisfaction of participants – except those who are especially fond of airing their opinions! It is easiest to continue with the present form of meetings without review, but this is an area where those who want to practise evidence-based management should be collecting and reviewing evidence of how effective and efficient the meetings in their organisation are.

Leadership and decision making

Clarity about who is leading the decision process helps implementation, but that does not tell us what kind of person is likely to be needed to lead different kinds of decisions. In so far as there is any choice, it is useful to think about the kind of decision and who would be most suitable to take a lead. Two forms of uncertainty make decisions more difficult to reach: one is uncertainty about the ends because of disagreements about what kind of outcome is preferable; the other is uncertainty about means. This means there are four different situations, each of which requires a different kind of leader.

- Where there is agreement about the desired outcome, and the means to get there are clear, an administrator can effectively take charge of ensuring that the process of reaching a decision goes logically through the different stages of the decision process. If this is done well it can be a good illustration of evidence-based management.
- Where there is a lot of uncertainty about the means, participants need to reach an agreement about what seems to be the best way forward, so a leader who can build consensus is wanted.

- Where there is disagreement about outcomes there has to be bargaining and negotiation, so a leader who is good at organisational politics is required.
- Where there is uncertainty about both ends and means choosing any course of action becomes almost impossible, so acting on hunch is the only possibility and for this to gain acceptance a charismatic leader is necessary.[15]

Using a different kind of leader for different types of decision is one way to try to improve the effectiveness of decision making, but it may not be practicable. Fortunately research has shown that managers vary their style according to the kind of decision, using participative approaches for decisions of most importance to subordinates and using them least for decisions of importance to the company.[16] A more directive approach can be appropriate in some circumstances, such as severe time constraints or where the subordinates do not know enough to contribute to a particular decision, but in general participation is more likely to help implementation.

Summary

There is a lot of research into decision making that can be useful in improving it. Decision making can usefully be analysed in terms of its stages and what can go wrong at each stage. It is often political as well as analytical, so part of the analysis necessary may be of the political interests involved in the decision and their relative power. Much of the research is about improving the process of decision making and is analytical in approach. But intuition can also be important in decision making and its value should be recognised and used. Two case studies illustrate how long-standing problems have been successfully tackled.

The main lessons from the research into decision making are summed up in the next section.

How to improve decision making

General

- Take decisions as far down in the organisation as possible, because people feel more motivated to implement decisions they have made or helped to make.
- Make it clear who is leading the decision process.
- Check whether you have agreed the objectives before starting on a decision process.
- Recognise that decision making rarely goes straight through the different stages of reaching a decision but often cycles back, so accept the ambiguity and uncertainty that brings, which is better than reaching the wrong decision.
- Beware of reaching a decision too quickly, asking whether too narrow a view has been taken of the problem.
- Decision making and evaluation should be linked. Build research into your decision making by making predictions about the results of the decision and the expected outcomes, and set up a system to collect and monitor the information that will tell you whether the decision is working out as expected. Do not wait until the end to assess progress.
- Remember the danger of remaining committed to a major decision, and spending more money and time, when it is going wrong. Be ready to examine the value of withdrawing before committing even further.

A good project for one of your staff taking an MBA is to examine decisions, either past or ongoing, to see how well they accord with the points above. Another project is to compare the subjects that have come up for decisions with those in a similar organisation as a check on what kind of subjects are being considered. Are there important subjects that you are not considering or ones on which a disproportionate amount of time is spent?

Problem identification

- How do you learn about problems?
- Do you have reliable systems to warn you of problems in all necessary areas?
- How well are these working? Are there examples of warnings that have been ignored?
- Are there problems that are being neglected? For what reasons? Are these still valid reasons? What are the tests of validity?
- Do you try to make sure you are tackling the right problem? To do so you may first need to understand the history of the problem: the when, what, where, who, how and why, before tackling the question of what should be done now.

Searching for a solution

- Examine what several organisations are doing about this and take what you think are the best features from each. In the public services, Beacons can make this easier than before.
- Identify more than one option for solution to avoid being trapped in a poor choice and not wanting to start again.
- Beware those who want to redefine the problem so that they can adopt a favourite solution, which is a particular danger in public policy.
- Where a parallel has been, or should be, drawn from the present problem to a previous one, listing the likenesses and the differences can help to show where the analogy may be misleading.
- There are other questions that will be relevant in examining solutions to some problems, such as: 'What are the measurable costs?', 'What are the measurable benefits?'

- Set up a devil's advocate for any major decision whose task it is to say why the course of action proposed may be wrong.

Implementation

- Start the preparation for implementation in the early stages.
- Early in the decision process seek to convince others about the need for action; enlisting their participation can be an effective way to do this.

Intuition is valuable too. While improving your evidence base also seek to cultivate your intuition.

These are individual points for improvement. But you should also make a more general check on your decision making by reviewing and evaluating a major decision in which you were involved. If it has not been successful try to identify where it went wrong. Do the same with another decision and ask yourself whether this suggests that there may be common weaknesses in decision making. If so, decide what can be done to reduce them.

Remember that your local university is likely to have students who need to do projects. They can be a useful resource in following up some of the analyses suggested above.

References

1 Falk R (1961) *The Business of Management: art or craft?* Penguin, Harmondsworth, p. 28.
2 McCall MW, Kaplan RE (1985) *Whatever It Takes: decision makers at work.* Prentice-Hall, Englewood Cliffs, NJ, p. 107.

3 Miller SJ, Hickson DJ, Wilson DA (1997) Decision-making in organisations. In: S Clegg, C Hardy and W Nord (eds) *Handbook of Organisation Studies*. Sage, New York. This gives a good overview of research into decision making.

4 Burns JM (1978) *Leadership*. Harper & Row, London.

5 Daker-White G, Carr AJ, Harvey I *et al.* (1999) A randomised control trial. Shifting boundaries of doctors and physiotherapists in orthopaedic outpatient departments. *J Epidemiol Community Health*. **53**: 643–50

6 Nutt PC (1999) Surprising but true: half the decisions in organisations fail. *Acad Mgmt Exec*. **13**(4): 75–90.

7 Butler RJ, Davies L, Pike R, Sharp J (1993) *Strategic Investment Decisions: theory, practice and process*. Routledge, London.

8 Janis IL, Mann L (1977) *Decision-making: a psychological analysis of conflict, choice and commitment*. Free Press, New York and Collier Macmillan, London.

9 *ibid.*, pp. 399–400.

10 Burke LA (1999) Taking the mystery out of intuitive decision-making. *Acad Mgmt Exec*. **13**(4): 91–9.

11 Isenberg DJ (1984) How senior managers think? *Harvard Business Review*. **84**(6): 81–90.

12 Hickson D, Butler RJ, Cray D *et al.* (1986) *Top Decisions: strategic decision-making in organisations*. Blackwell, Oxford.

13 *ibid.*, p. 250.

14 Butler RJ (1996) Decision-making. In: M Warner (ed.) *International Encyclopedia of Business and Management*. Routledge, London.

15 *ibid.*, p. 965.

16 Bass BB (1990) *Bass & Stogdill's Handbook of Leadership: theory, research and managerial applications* (3e). Free Press, New York and Collier Macmillan, London, pp. 442–3.

6

Learning to practise evidence-based management

Be willing to think that you may be wrong, unlike a surgeon's comment on his colleagues: 'Often wrong, but never in doubt'.

The aim of this chapter is to describe what managers need to learn to practise evidence-based management, what are the problems of doing so, and who and what can help their learning. Therefore it has a specific focus; managers who also want a more general account of how to learn and how to improve organisational learning can find that in the large literature on the subject.[1]

What needs to be learnt

What you need to learn to practise evidence-based management depends on what you already know – 'knowing' includes being able to do. Many of the learning needs should be clear from the previous chapters and the ways of improving suggested at the end of each chapter. What you may need to learn to do is to:

- manage the job to make time and space to improve performance
- recognise your mental map – how you make sense of the world
- make use of those who see things differently
- question your and others' assumptions
- check the reliability of evidence
- access good sources of information efficiently
- make use of intuitive knowledge as well as analytical
- ask searching questions about performance and research the answers
- be alert to what needs monitoring
- ensure that the monitoring is reliable
- improve your decision making.

An important part of learning is also knowing what to discard. Much of that happens unconsciously as we become more skilled and knowledgeable, but it can still be very useful to take stock occasionally of our work habits and our beliefs. Many of the workshops provided by consultants and management training centres are aimed to help managers improve their work habits. The most long-standing examples are the workshops on time management and quicker reading; both can be useful for those who want to practise evidence-based management. Reviewing our beliefs is more of a challenge: it is discussed below in the section on assumptions.

An article on evidence-based management argues that one of the obstacles to its practice is that managers are not trained or experienced in the use of empirical evidence in making management decisions.[2] Management educators might disagree, arguing that the use of case studies is the way of doing just this. However, the article comes from the US, where proportionately more people take MBAs and more hospital managers have degrees in health management than in the UK, so the criticism is likely to be even more applicable in the UK. If it is – and readers should ask themselves whether they agree – then the learning problem is to develop the mind-set that asks: 'What is the evidence?', 'How good is it?', 'How can we check it?' and 'What can we do to get the evidence that we require?'.

Knowing when one needs to learn

You may easily recognise some learning needs, such as improving your use of the Internet or problem analysis; others that are more important may not be recognised, because they require an insight into your ways of thinking and working. It is difficult to recognise when change is needed because research suggests that we notice what we expect, so our expectations are self-confirming, and we ration-alise isolated contradictions as exceptions that do not merit attention.[3] We see what we expect to see.

The problem is how to become aware of your, and your group's, errors and remediable limitations. There are two main ways of doing so. One is to try to do it for yourself, for which the most helpful technique is reflective practice. The other is feedback from others. The most useful idea for evidence-based management from all the theoretical writing on reflective practice is the importance of learning from reflecting on what we do so that we can improve our practice. Johns, writing for nurses, listed questions as a guide to learning, which are also useful for other professions.[4] Simple ways of reflecting on what happened and what you could do to improve are given in the 'How to improve' section at the end of this chapter.

Feedback is the second way of learning what you need to change in your own work or in that of the organisation. A good staff appraisal scheme can be very helpful, provided it is done well, but too many managers shirk giving a real appraisal or are too unskilled to do it well. Accurate feedback from the staff can be difficult to get because people do not like to give unwelcome news. But it can be very helpful: I remember when I was a young newly promoted manager of a small research organisation and an older woman said to me: 'You should say "thank you" more often!'. I hated the comment, but it taught me to be more appreciative of what staff did and to show that appreciation. One reason why managers often do not get the feedback they need is because, as whistle-blowers have found, it often gets them into trouble and may not improve the situation.

Another good source of feedback on performance is from the users. Some organisations, particularly some companies, regard this as a crucially important guide to their performance. Toyota, for example, sends recent buyers of one of its cars a most detailed questionnaire about their experience in buying and using the car. The response provides a way of measuring customer satisfaction. Many businesses, like Toyota, use the analysis of customer reactions as a way of learning what may be going wrong with the product or in the service delivery.

In the public sector, the views of users usually receive less attention, unless there is a formal complaint. However, the attitude of at least some public services has been changing; noteworthy is the Inland Revenue's provision of a telephone helpline for filling in the tax return, which is available when the offices are closed, including weekends. This is not a source of feedback, except perhaps for what taxpayers find difficult, but does reflect more concern for the public. In the NHS, there is a danger that the drive to involve patients may be seen as an imposed duty, rather than a valuable form of feedback about how services are actually working.

It can be particularly hard for a cohesive group to learn other ways of thinking because cohesiveness encourages conformity: a desire not to rock the boat or risk the unpopularity that can come from opposing accepted ideas. It is easier if the whole group wants to learn; there are some things you can learn on your own but others, particularly those affecting group decision making, that require support from at least some members of the group. You may need to proselytise as well as to overcome your own temptation to follow old habits rather than developing new and better ones.

Learning to recognise and test assumptions

'Mental maps' is a good metaphor to explain that we all have our own ways of observing and interpreting what is happening. We make assumptions, often unconsciously, about what is important. These assumptions determine how we seek to explain what has happened and what we should do next.

One of the most vivid examples of how different assumptions and ways of viewing the world can affect the explanations offered for what is going on was provided by Allison[5] in his account of different explanations for the Cuban missile crisis (when there was an imminent threat of war between the USA and the Soviet Union, as it then was, because the Soviet Union had placed missiles on Cuba which could directly threaten the USA). Allison presents his account as a way of showing that how we explain things, and how we make decisions, depends on the categories we use and the assumptions we make. This is a real-life case and, at the time, a crucially important detective story, because what the protagonists did depended on their views of what the other was doing, and hence the chances of a catastrophic war. Each of Allison's three accounts of what happened and why sounds convincing, but they reach very different conclusions about what was going on. They do this because in trying to explain what happened, they asked different questions and so looked for different kinds of evidence and came up with different explanations. To the reader who has not read the other explanations, each analysis sounds convincing, because within its own assumptions it makes sense.

The first analysis, called the Rational Actor, which is the most commonly used, starts from the assumption that if you are trying to answer the question 'Why did the Soviet government decide to install missiles in Cuba?', it can be explained if it can be shown to be a reasonable action given Soviet strategic objectives, so these are what must be analysed. The other two explanations start from what we have learnt about how organisations actually work: that any organisation, including a government, is composed of many different interests and skills with different approaches to problems, so that unified, coherent action is very hard to achieve. Also cockups can occur because of deficiencies in the organisational systems and the different objectives and working methods of different parts of the organisation. So to explain the Soviet actions you need to look at what actually happened and try to understand why it happened like that by examining the ways in which the Soviet military organisation actually works. Hence an analysis that is only based on what would be the rational thing to do, given Soviet strategic objectives, will be inadequate.

The lesson that emerges from this and other studies is that even when an analysis sounds convincing you should explore how it would look if different assumptions were made. It would have been much harder for those caught up in the Cuban missile crisis to have done so, because that would have required a different way of thinking about how organisations actually work. Are they, for example, controlled by the leader at the top? If that is the working assumption then it is understanding the leader's views and objectives that matters. Or are there different organisational groups with their own interests and systems which will affect what actually happens? Such a view would require a different kind of analysis to explain what was happening. How well do the organisational systems for the delivery of top decisions actually work? Once that question is asked, there is a possibility that a cock-up may be part, at least, of the explanation of what was going on.

We have to limit what we are looking at when we are trying to understand a problem and reach a decision. The most common ways of doing so, often unconsciously, is to set boundaries, start from a reference point or perspective and select the way(s) of measuring success or failure. It is hard to recognise the boundaries you use, which you have learnt from your training and cultural background. A useful learning exercise to help you recognise and appraise the way you seek to limit decision making is to examine a particular decision – either on your own or as a group exercise – and ask what assumptions were made, what was taken for granted and whether that was appropriate. For example, whether a recent expenditure on a new piece of equipment was described in terms of how it could save money or in terms of what it would cost and whether the other way of describing it could have affected the decision.

Your reference point or perspective also affects how you view a decision. Are you optimistic or pessimistic? How urgent or important do you think it is? Learning to consider alternative perspectives from the one you usually adopt is a good way of improving your decision making. Some managers, for example, have a greater sense of urgency than others, or are parsimonious, and will use one or both as reference points, whether it is necessary or not.

How an outcome is measured can also influence reactions to the figures; whether it is described in percentages or actual amounts can affect judgement of the outcome and the decision that is reached. For example, which measure you use in telling your manager that you are over budget can influence how he or she judges this. Similarly in describing the extra money that is needed for a project that is already over budget a percentage of a large sum may seem less than the actual figure.

Sources of learning

Learning from your own experience

Most people probably think it is useful to learn from their own experience, both of what has gone well and, perhaps even more importantly, from what has gone badly. Reflective practice is one way of learning to improve your own practice, but there are other ways for individuals and groups to learn from their experience. Yet this happens too rarely in organisations unless special steps are taken to stimulate and facilitate such learning. The managing director who did not recognise a case study of one of his company's new product failures, mentioned in Chapter 3, is an example of someone who paid attention to successes – he recognised the case study of a successful new product – but not to failures, so was not able to learn from them. Even when there are inquiries into disasters in the public sector they may not ensure that the lessons drawn from what went wrong are remembered or that the necessary changes are actually made to prevent it happening again. As the report *An Organisation with a Memory* about learning from adverse incidents in the NHS, described on p. 89, points out:

> *Too often lessons are identified but true 'active' learning does not take place because the necessary changes are not properly embedded in practice. . . .*
>
> *The time is right for a fundamental re-thinking of the way that the NHS approaches the challenge of learning from adverse health care events. The NHS often fails to learn the lessons when things go wrong, and has an old-fashioned approach in this area compared to some other sectors.*[6]

They go on to say:

> *The NHS does not, in our experience, learn effectively*

and actively from failures. Too often, valid lessons are drawn from adverse events but their implementation throughout the NHS is very patchy. Active learning is mostly confined to the organisation in which the adverse event occurs. The NHS is **par excellence** *a passive learning organisation.*[7]

If you want to learn from experience, and any reader of this book should want to do so, then there are methods of making organisational learning easier. One is to have an after-action review (AAR). The US Army was the first large organisation to introduce AARs: there is a hot review, during the action, and a cold one immediately after. AARs are now used in some large US companies. They would be equally useful in the public sector.

Five simple questions are used to guide the discussion.

- What was the intent?
- What happened? This question should be asked as soon as possible when it is easier to remember what happened.
- What was learned?
- What do we do now?
- Who else should we tell?

Half an hour to an hour can be long enough to gain insights into what to do.[8] The discipline of doing so regularly can encourage individuals and groups to reflect on and to share what they have learned from this.

There is a motivational problem to learning from experience; it requires you to be wrong some of the time. Mistakes may be punished either directly or by loss of the prestige from success. This is why feedback of the results of organisational action is often distorted or suppressed, or arrives after the need for learning as a basis for changing the action has passed.[9] To try to encourage reliable feedback of mistakes and performance problems, the aim should be to create an atmosphere where mistakes, including decisions that have gone wrong, are treated as a good source of learning by the manager in coaching subordinates and by reviews within the group that made a mistaken decision.

Learning from others' experience

It may seem easier, and more ego enhancing, to make your own decisions about what to do and how to tackle a new government requirement than to check on what others are doing. Hopefully – but research is needed to check whether this is so – the greater ease in finding information via the Web and the development of Beacons (*see* pp. 63–4) in various parts of the public sector will change this approach. It should also encourage a much wider interest in discovering what others are doing, or have done.

The experience of others can be helpful in two different ways: one, to learn how they have tackled a similar problem and two, perhaps less commonly, as a stimulus for thinking about how to tackle a problem. There are problem areas which may arouse feelings of concern, but where you may have no clear ideas about how to tackle them. The evidence-based manager will seek out examples in other organisations where the problem has been tackled successfully. For example, one such area may be the special health and social problems of ethnic populations. One example given in Chapter 4 was of the circumstances of Yemeni elders. Another example of a distinctive approach to tackling this is the Asian Cookery Club Project in Bedfordshire and Luton Community NHS Trust.

Box 6.1:   Asian Cookery Club

This project is of interest for three reasons.
 • It is an example of a successful development with a good concern

for evidence at all stages, although one with problems, acknowledged by the organiser, of doing a satisfactory evaluation. The
target group offers particular challenges as it is difficult to access
and there are language difficulties in communication.

- It has been active and developing since 1995. Funding has come
from Bedfordshire Health Authority (years 1 and 2), the British
Heart Foundation (year 3) and in the past two years, Luton
Health Action Zone (HAZ). The project received Beacon status in
1999 for two years.
- It is an unusually popular Beacon site, even though it is not
dealing with one of the usual NHS concerns.

Background
The project was initiated in 1995 by a community dietitian from
South Bedfordshire Community Healthcare Trust, under the
umbrella of the Bedfordshire Food Strategy. This is a multi-agency
alliance aiming to help the population of Bedfordshire to have a
healthier diet. Of particular concern was the greater risk of
coronary heart disease and diabetes in the South Asian communities and the difficulties of accessing and working with these
groups. In Luton, where 20% of the population is from the South
Asian continent, a priority was seen to be to identify a way of
working with the community to address these health problems.

A literature review at the time showed that most of the research
about the South Asian communities was about the access to healthcare and whether the care available was culturally acceptable.
There was very little about any practical initiatives for addressing
health promotion around diet.

The idea of using cookery clubs was suggested as a means of
conveying healthy eating advice, specifically around reduction of
fats, in a practical, culturally acceptable way to the South Asian
communities.

The clubs were focused on the women of the community, as it
was thought that they would then be able to take the dietary
messages home and introduce them into their family's diet.

Aim
To encourage members of the Asian community in the use of
healthier recipes and healthy cooking techniques in everyday living.

Objectives
- To introduce culturally acceptable healthy eating.
- To encourage and develop healthier cooking skills.
- To allow social interaction.

As the project has developed the objectives have adapted to meet the changing needs.

Current outcomes
- To provide accredited training for all cookery club leaders at Level 2 with the National Open College Network in 'Community Nutrition Skills' and 'Being a Cookery Club Leader Skills'.
- To provide accredited training at Level 3 for all club leaders while they are running clubs.
- To sustain cookery clubs in Luton.
- To provide regular support to the team of 11 cookery club leaders.
- To develop appropriate evaluation tools.

Method
In the early years of the project, the clubs were facilitated by Look After Yourself Tutors, but later the women from the local community were recruited and trained to do this.

Each club leader recruits 10–12 local women who share the same first language, Urdu, Gujarati or Bengali, to attend a cookery club. There are five sessions in one club programme: an introductory session, three of practical cookery and a reunion party used for evaluation.

During the cookery sessions the women work together in small groups preparing and cooking traditional dishes. At the end of the session the women taste the dishes and discuss their thoughts. The cookery club leader facilitates the whole experience. The women are encouraged to take the recipes home and try the healthier cooking techniques in their homes.

Challenges
The project has faced many challenges over the years, which are discussed in the annual reports and the Asian Cookery Club Process Notes.

Particular concerns in working with community women as club leaders have been their ability to commit to the project and issues about their payment. Their requirements for training and support are high. Finding suitable venues has also been a problem.

Evaluation
Each year of the project there has been a different focus to the evaluation. In the earlier years, the emphasis was on the suitability of the training pack and the training given to the club leaders. In addition, information was collected from the women on dietary changes they made at home.

A more elaborate evaluation was possible in 1999/2000 because of funding from the Luton HAZ. For the first time, evaluation was focused on the club leaders as well as the participants. The community dietitian's observation of the club leaders while running their clubs proved very informative and led to the development of a more comprehensive training programme, which provides the club leaders with an accreditation. Club leaders were also encouraged to record their reflections of their clubs and feed these back to the dietitian.

The feedback from the club participants has been gathered using a semi-structured questionnaire, usually collected by the community dietitian. When necessary, one of the women in the group was used as an interpreter.

Many women reported making changes to their diet as a result of coming to the clubs. Many also reported desirable weight loss. There was, however, a marked difference between the Gujarati women, who were more likely to be able to make changes at home, and the Bangladeshi women, who found their families more resistant to change. Some women with diabetes said that if they could not change the family's meal they cooked separately for themselves after attending the club. None of the women was willing to offer guests the healthier eating recipes when they entertained.

The organiser, the community dietitian, has questioned the evaluation tools used to collect feedback on dietary changes and said that it 'has been particularly problematic, due to the abilities of the club leaders and the language limitations of the target group'.

In evidence-based management, it is important to recognise the desirability of evaluation, but also what factors limit its reliability.

It was noted by some women that men had to be involved in the project if changes in cooking at home were to be accepted.

In the fifth year of the project, an accredited training programme with National Open College Network was developed for all club leaders. It was identified that if the club leaders were to be working independently in the community, it was vital that their under-standing of the key nutrition messages and their ability to deliver the clubs was assessed. These credits will be available for other trainers to access and the training materials and assessment tools will be available to purchase.

Since the delivery of the first accredited course for the club leaders, a full review of the training has been written.

There has been a lot of interest in the project, especially since gaining Beacon status in 1998, with its own website and money to organise learning visits. There have been 12 Beacon visits bringing together people doing or thinking about doing similar kinds of project work, with a database of 170 people.

Diabetes cookery clubs
An adapted programme specifically for South Asian people with diabetes was made possible by money from Partnership for Change (Department of Health Funding). The work was developed with the same group of cookery club leaders using a similar programme; the main difference was the referral method, usually from health professionals. However, a final report found that it was not successful for a number of reasons, including the referral procedure, the need for blood tests, insufficient training of the club leaders and the stigma associated with diabetes in the South Asian community.

Further information and copies of reports can be obtained from stephanie.cash@ldh-tr.anglox.nhs.uk

A very different kind of Beacon, but one which also has a heavy emphasis on how to do it, is Nottingham City Hospital NHS Trust's development of competency schemes.

Box 6.2: Development of competency schemes in Nottingham City Hospital NHS Trust

This case study is included because it is an example of:
- the time and care spent in developing competencies as a guide to appraisal and training needs analysis
- details of the Beacon learning activities and their evaluation, which is a requirement of a Beacon award and helps to provide evidence of the reported utility of learning provided by the Beacon.

Background
Work on the development of competencies started in 1992/93 using behavioural event and critical incident techniques to describe effective senior manager and executive director competencies. The work on further development was greatly assisted by the acquisition of the MEDEQUATE competence modeller in 1995/96. This programme generates generic competencies for posts and was a useful starting point for work in theatres and oncology, and has been taken forward to become the generic nursing competencies and competencies for other staff such as medical secretaries and chaplains.

Its recognition as a Beacon and the only HR Nye Bevan award, has been the link between this work, training needs analysis, personal development planning and appraisal, and true staff involvement as fundamental for the management of change.

Beacon dissemination and evaluation
The Beacon award was received in July 1999 for two years, and the HR Nye Bevan award provided individual bursaries to trust staff with the aim of spreading best practice.

The visit programme has consisted of 10 full-day 'visits' to the trust and six half-day bespoke sessions for 130 people from over 30 trusts, including seven entire Directorate teams. This is more events than any other HR Beacon.

This programme has been supported by a team of seven senior staff from oncology, theatres and human resources.

Other dissemination has included: over 200 special Beacon packs, ad hoc enquiries, conference attendance and presentations.

Learning has been seen as two-way, because of the opportunity provided to learn from others' experience.

Evaluation ratings have been high, including answers to the questions: 'Will this visit prompt you to initiate change in your organisation?' Two individual criticisms are relevant to evidence-based management: 'lack of hard data on costing' and 'lack of hard evidence but counterbalanced by enthusiasm'. Otherwise the evaluation comments were positive.

The enthusiasm referred to, exemplified by the involvement of senior staff in the Beacon programmes, is evidence of the perceived success of the programme, even though there was no 'hard evidence', but it may be difficult to prove the connection between the competency programme and subsequent changes. The questions form part of the Theatre Competency Progression Scheme Personal Profile, with sections called 'Evidence of', and should encourage a consideration in the appraisal interview of the evidence provided in this profile.

Such easily accessible facilities as Beacons for learning from others may change what managers do. Whether they do will depend on:

- how well the managers manage their job so that they have time and interest to try to improve
- whether they see learning from others as a way of doing so
- how they think and, in particular, whether they want to practise evidence-based management.

There is also the danger, discussed in Chapter 3, of inertia, so that the knowledge gained does not get translated into action.

An often-neglected source of good ideas for improvement is the views of more junior grades of staff. Suggestion schemes are the traditional way to tap these and, imaginatively run, they can be useful. Southwest Airlines in the US has shown that the traditional way can be improved by being made much less formal. Employees are encouraged to take ideas to anyone in the company whom they believe can evaluate them for effectiveness. Employees are said to know from experience that their ideas will get attention, assessment and a response. Several media are used to publicise new ideas from staff, including print publications, intranet and videos played on company TVs. Suggestions outside an employee's immediate work area are encouraged by cross-functional meetings aimed at helping staff understand the wider operations.[10]

Learning from the past

There can be a similar but even greater problem in learning from the past than in learning from others: it takes more effort, and if the source of learning is, or has to be, acknowledged, carries much less kudos than developing your own ideas. One of the striking aspects of organisations in the public and private sectors is the neglect of the experience of earlier managers in similar jobs, even where previous practice was better than the present. Nor does the explanation seem to be simply the result of staff turnover and no or poor records of previous practice, although these are part of the problem. This neglect of previous experience seems particularly true of staff jobs, and of those in policy jobs, perhaps because their incumbents feel a special need to prove their worth by developing their own ideas.*

Some previous work and experience ceases to be relevant because of the many changes, but many of the problems,

---

*A thought-provoking and practical book about how US policy makers could, but failed to, learn from history, with practical suggestions for other decision makers, is Neustadt RE, May ER (1986) *Thinking in Time: the uses of history for decision makers*. Free Press, New York.

such as the management of outpatient departments, remain similar to those in the past. It is depressing to find on visiting a hospital, or the management training department of a large company, that no one knows about earlier achievements or would be interested in them if they did. It seems that able and dedicated people make improvements, but when they leave these decay. This could be partly the loss of their leadership skills, but good leadership should leave behind people who are interested and able to continue good performance and who want to improve still more.

The practice of evidence-based management should help to reduce, if not remedy, this neglect of previous experience by: first, encouraging an interest in looking for evidence, including evidence of what was done before, and in learning from it, and second, developing records of what is being done that can be available to, and useful for, those who come after. The latter is a subject of great interest to information technologists who want to capture organisational memory. This is much easier for information technologists to do for some purposes than for others. Codifiable expertise can be captured, as it is for doctors and for consultants in Accenture, who have developed an intranet site called Knowledge Space, which has a variety of information, including global best practices, that a consultant in the field can access. It is harder to capture in databases the expertise that is a mix of explicit and tacit knowledge, as is true for much expertise.

There is another problem in expecting databases to provide the main answer to capturing organisational memory: it is that managers rely more on their network for information and advice. People are said to be about five times more likely to turn to other people for answers than to other sources of information: 'who you know significantly affects what you eventually know'.[11] Working together on a project team or participating in the same management course can increase people's knowledge for that reason, as well as by what they learn individually while doing so. This social aspect of information sharing and mutual learning needs to be considered in setting up project teams.

Making use of lessons from the past is achieved in a variety of ways. A US study of learning from 22 projects in different kinds of company showed the ways in which learning from these projects was remembered. These were:

- in the minds of individual employees
- in the relationships that are used for ongoing work
- in databases and filing cabinets
- in work processes
- in the products and services that have developed from previous experience.[11]

It is, the authors suggest, the lessons from one-time events that may not be captured unless there is a systematic attempt to do so. This is where the AARs, described earlier in this chapter, are useful. Much of the organisational memory resides in individuals and therefore is at greatest risk of being lost to the organisation if that individual leaves. This is particularly marked where that person played a key role in the social interaction around a task where much learning can take place, as can be true in many project teams and in clinical teams. A debrief interview and a final group discussion seeking to highlight what the group has learnt can be ways of reducing the loss.

Learning from research

This cannot be such an important source of learning in management as in medicine, for the reasons discussed in Chapter 1, but it can and should be a more important one than it is in many organisations. There are many opportunities for research apart from the most expensive one of commissioning research, although that can be worthwhile too. There is already published research; an example was given in Chapter 3 of the use of social research as a guide to reducing the human problems of mergers. This book has drawn heavily on published research that has useful lessons for those wanting to practise evidence-based management. There is the research done in-house, good examples of which were given in Chapter 1. Now that more managers and clinicians are taking Masters degrees, which require them to do a field project, they offer a useful opportunity for extra research resources. Finally, a responsive attitude to research groups wanting to do part of their fieldwork in your organisation can be very rewarding because, apart from any useful findings, the questions the researchers ask can stimulate you to think afresh about what you are doing.

Lifelong learning

This can be seen in different ways. In France, it is seen as an entitlement for every citizen. In the UK, continuous professional development (CPD) is a well-recognised need for professionals prescribed by their professional bodies. The Engineering Council described its nature well, when in 1997 they made CPD a requirement for the first time:

> *The systematic maintenance, improvement and broadening of knowledge, understanding and skill, and the development of personal qualities necessary for the execution of professional and technical duties throughout the individual's working life.*[12]

Another description, by Houle, offers a more personal commitment, which is applicable to managers in the public sector:

> *The ways in which professionals try, throughout their*

active lives of service, to refresh their own knowledge and ability and build a sense of collective responsibility to society.[13]

But there is no equivalent requirement or even commonly accepted aspiration for managers. One reason is that there is no required educational qualification for managers, yet managers also need to keep up to date with all the changes affecting their jobs and to be stimulated to think critically about how they work. There is a widespread recognition in large organisations, both public and private, that there is a need for further education for managers, particularly when moving to a more senior level. There are also different policies and initiatives to encourage learning, as the idea of the learning organisation has become fashionable. So in most large organisations, including the NHS, there is encouragement for further learning.

Managers interested in practising evidence-based management should accept the need for lifelong learning, believing that they should always be seeking to improve and that the ability to think critically needs to be stimulated and developed. They should seek to ensure that the knowledge they acquire is evidence based, which will give them a special interest in learning about the findings of new research studies relevant to their work. It should also give them an interest in critically appraising how they work, to provide the evidence about what they actually do as distinct from what they believe they do.

The prime obstacle to managers pursuing CPD is the pressures on them, so that a supportive culture is particularly important. In the next chapter we shall look at what this is and what the manager can do to help develop it.

Summary

The aim of this chapter, summarised on the first page, was to help you to recognise what you may need to learn if you are to practise evidence-based management successfully. Most important is to value and use evidence, if you do not already do so. Some learning needs will be easy to recognise, others are harder because they require an understanding of how you think and work. Learning to identify your own and others' assumptions is hard, so some of the suggestions below will be helpful.

It helps to make good use of all the sources of learning: your own experience, other people's practice, research and the past, both for the good examples and for the lessons from past failings.

How to improve

- Seek to learn from what happens by having reviews of action, asking questions like 'What was the aim?', 'What actually happened?', 'What did we learn?', 'Are there changes that we should make as a result of that learning?'. Make sure you allow time for this rather than pressing on. Such reviews can usefully be applied to important meetings and major decisions as well as to the handling of an emergency or a recent reorganisation.
- Practise learning to examine assumptions. Particularly when an analysis sounds convincing, check to see how it would look with different assumptions. To do this you have to be able to recognise what assumptions have been made. An aid to doing this is to classify the information that you are using into three columns: known, unclear, presumed. Known information can be the basis for action, but there should be further search or only cautious action where the information is presumed or unclear.[14]
- Examine the assumptions made about learning needs. For example, take the topics listed in *NHS Beacon Services* and ask what that says about assumptions on learning.
- Make a special point of reviewing adverse incidents, if this is not already done.

- Encourage honest feedback from staff, both of your own work and manner and of performance in your unit.
- Get feedback from users about all aspects of performance.
- Reward people for thoughtful analyses of problems and solutions.
- An old, but still useful, idea for capturing employees' knowledge and ideas is the suggestion scheme. It is likely to work best when there is a group to evaluate the ideas – in Xerox this is called the Tiger Team, and the service engineers who make most good suggestions are made a member of this team, which is a highly valued position.[15]
- An even better idea is to develop the welcoming approach to new ideas used by Southwest Airlines in the US, described above.
- Keep a journal of critical incidents; when you are a new professional try to do this daily. Later a weekly journal would still be a good way to reflect on what you do and how you could improve. Useful headings for analysis are: Description, what happened? How you felt about it? Evaluation: good and bad? Analysis: how do you explain it? Conclusion: what else could you have done? What would you do next time?
- Review what you do to keep up to date and to be mentally stimulated and ask yourself what form of learning works best for you? Is there a gap between your intentions and what you actually do? If so, how can you bridge it?

References

1 Pedler M, Burgoyne J, Boydell T (1991) *The Learning Company: a strategy for sustainable development*. McGraw-Hill, Maidenhead. A practical book with many useful suggestions.
Davies H, Nutley S (2000) Developing learning organisations in the New NHS. *BMJ*. **320**: 998–1001. This

gives a useful summary of the points made by the leading academic writers on organisational learning.

2 Kovner A, Elton J, Billings J *et al.* (2000) Evidence-based management/commentaries/reply. *Front Health Serv Mgmt*. **16**(4): 3–46.

3 Feldman J (1986) On the difficulty of learning from experience. In: H Sims Jr, D Gioia *et al.* (eds) *The Thinking Organization*. Jossey-Bass, San Francisco, CA.

4 Johns C (1994) Nuances of reflection. *J Clin Nurs*. **3**: 71–5.

5 Allison G (1971) *The Essence of Decision: explaining the Cuban missile crisis*. Little, Brown & Co., Boston, MA.

6 Department of Health (2000) *An Organisation with a Memory*. The Stationery Office, London, p. xi.

7 *ibid.*, pp. 77–8.

8 Cross R, Baird L (2000) Technology is not enough: improving performance by building organizational memory. *Sloan Mgmt Rev*. **41**(3): 69–78.

9 Huber G (1991) Organizational learning: the contributing processes and the literatures. *Org Sci*: **2**: 195.

10 Frontline Knowledge (2000) Idea-sharing at Southwest Airlines. *Knowl Mgmt Rev*. **3**(1): 3.

11 Cross R, Baird L, *op. cit.*, p. 72.

12 Engineering Council (1997) *Standards and Routes to Registration* (SARTOR) (3e). The Engineering Council, London, p. 29.

13 Houle C (1980) *Continuing Learning in the Professions*. Jossey-Bass, San Francisco, CA.

14 Neustadt R, May E (1986) *Thinking in Time: the uses of history for decision makers*. Free Press, New York.

15 Cross R, Baird L, *op. cit.*, p. 76.

7

Organisational culture

The NHS culture is not – by and large – one which encourages reporting and analysis.[1]

The Trust aims to achieve a culture in which clinical excellence and high quality is central to service delivery. We recognise that this will only be achieved in a learning culture, not one of blame so that quality is integral to all aspects of the Trust's work. This includes the willingness to embrace constructive criticism and new ideas as well as a determination to break down any barriers which may exist.[2]

Organisations develop distinctive cultures because people working together tend, after a time, to think and act in similar ways. This fact matters for many aspects of management, but particularly in the management of change since the culture of the organisation, or that of powerful groups within it, may be opposed to change. The relevance of organisational culture for this book is that individuals in the organisation come to process and evaluate information in somewhat similar ways, for example in the importance they attach to evidence and in the kind of evidence that is valued. Managers interested in the practice of evidence-based management should ask themselves whether the culture is favourable to its practice and if not, what could be done to make it more so.

In any organisation, there can be, and usually are, a number of different cultures. There is the culture of the organisation as a whole, which in some organisations can be very strong. Marks and Spencer, for example, has had for a long time an unusually distinctive culture. This can be a source of great strength, as it was for that company for many years, but it can also make it harder to adapt to change. A strong culture may also encourage or discourage an evidence-based approach. The opening quotation above suggests that the culture of the NHS does not make it easy to practise evidence-based management.

There can also be distinctive cultures within an organisation, particularly in different professions and specialisms. In the NHS, there are marked distinctive cultures, with the medical culture being the most distinctive and having within it further distinctions, such as that between surgeons and general medicine or between GPs and hospital doctors. Strong cultures bind people together but in doing so make members of that culture self-protective and resistant to attempts by 'outsiders' to change them.

Sir Donald Irvine, president of the General Medical Council, the body responsible for doctors' self-regulation, made a strong criticism of the medical culture in a speech at the Royal Society of Medicine on 16 January 2001, saying:

> The cultural flaws in the medical profession show up as excessive paternalism, lack of respect for patients and their right to make decisions about their care, secrecy and complacency about poor practice.

What is the culture of your organisation?

A guide to whether the culture is favourable to the practice of evidence-based management is given by considering where

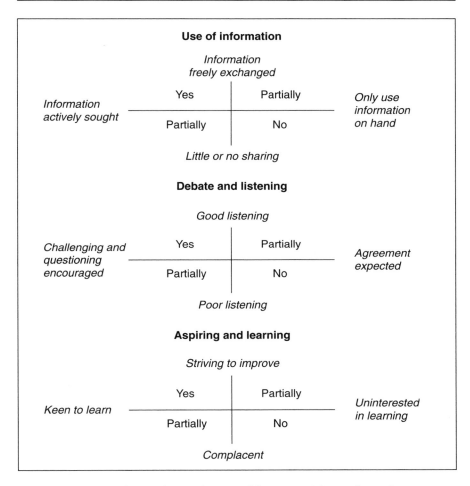

Figure 7.1   Is the culture favourable to evidence-based management?

the organisation belongs in each of the quadrants in Figure 7.1: the top left is best and the bottom right is worst.

A culture that encourages an active search for information is much more common in some types of organisation than in others.[3] In stockbroking, consulting and newspaper publishing staff are encouraged to seek information through personal contacts as well as written sources. This may then be shared with their colleagues to improve understanding of what is happening in the environment. The office and refreshment arrangements may be designed to encourage the sharing of information. The growth of the Internet, and the intranet (for internal exchanges), has provided another means of sharing information, but they do not eliminate the value of personal contact. In organisations that are less dependent for their success on their understanding of their environment, organisational culture may also encourage information sharing, though this can vary widely even within different parts of the same large organisation and between organisations in the same sector.

The proximity of GPs in a GP practice, and the fact that it is a partnership, should encourage active sharing of information, but there are wide differences between practices in the extent to which they share information and provide for this to happen on a regular basis. There are also considerable differences in whether they seek to share information with their patients and if so, in how they do this. The development of the NHS Beacon Services, which includes a high proportion of primary care practices, includes some examples of an active interest in obtaining and sharing information, like Cookham Medical Centre included in Chapter 4.

The culture will also influence whether a conflict of opinions is accepted and whether other people's views are listened to. In some organisations, there is a strong pressure to conform to accepted views and disagreement is frowned on, and a conflict of views even more so. Different views are either not listened to or only as a means of rebuttal, not as a potentially useful contribution to the discussion. The stronger the culture the greater the likelihood that disagreement will be discouraged, unless the culture is one that is supportive of evidence-based management. The research into group behaviour has shown how strong group pressures can be on individuals.

Research by Janis[4] first suggested that a highly cohesive

group could be dysfunctional for the effectiveness of the group. He coined the phrase 'group think' to describe this danger. He described the symptoms of group think as:

- a marked decrease in the openness of group members to discrepant or unsettling information because of the strong pressures towards uniformity
- simultaneous unwillingness to seriously examine such information when it is brought to the group's attention
- the avoidance of controversial issues.

He compared high- and low-quality decisions by policy-making groups and concluded that there were five conditions that contributed to group think:

- high cohesiveness
- insulation of the group
- lack of methodological procedures for search and appraisal
- directive leadership
- high stress and little hope of finding a better solution.

This list suggests that it is possible to retain the advantages of a cohesive group and to avoid its dangers if evidence-based management is practised in the ways described in earlier chapters, and the group is not insulated from external, and possibly divergent, views.

Whether there is a strong desire to improve and an eagerness to learn is another aspect of the culture that affects the ease of practising evidence-based management. Complacency is counter-productive, as a need for change will only be recognised when there is dissatisfaction with the status quo. Another danger is a culture of cynicism, as Graham Leicester describes it in an editorial to a series of articles on the role of evidence in public sector policy and practice:

This is the culture that allows us to go along with the 'company view' or the 'conventional wisdom', even when we know it to be false, since our professional lives and career advancement depend on maintaining the lie. We show that we are aware of the deception and therefore not tainted by it by sounding off about how ridiculous this way of operation is in the pub with colleagues after work, complaining about how senior management must be crazy if they think they are fooling anyone. But we do nothing to change it, or to challenge formally the 'company truth'.[5]

He describes this culture of cynicism as an aspect of civil service culture but also more widespread.

A more accurate way of assessing the culture than in the do-it-yourself diagrams given above is to conduct a survey that asks diagnostic questions about many aspects of the organisation. Such surveys will commonly use a rating scale from the most negative to the most positive. For example, survey items that would be relevant to evidence-based management include:

- How open and free is the flow of information? Do people express ideas and opinions easily and openly?
- To what extent are staff expected to conform to norms of behaviour, rules, procedures and policies or to think for themselves?
- How much are staff ideas, opinions and suggestions sought out, encouraged and valued?
- Are staff satisfied with their organisation's performance?

The survey could be conducted among the staff only or it could also be given to those in close contact with the organisation, which may provide a truer picture than that given by insiders. Another way of getting outsiders' views is to interest your local management school in sending their managerial students on a culture visit to you. Their task would be to describe what they noticed that was distinctive about how people behave in your organisation. It is remarkable how easy it is, with a little prior training, to notice cultural differences between organisations.

The values underlying evidence-based management

An aspect of the culture is the common values that people hold. The values that are needed for evidence-based management should have emerged from the previous chapters, but may still need crystallising. They can be summed up as beliefs in the values of:

- objectivity
- critical appraisal of evidence
- using, as far as practical, the best evidence available
- listening to other people's experience and opinions
- willingness to accept that you may be wrong
- willingness to share information
- an enthusiasm for learning from others' experience and from research.

But to be effective these need to be accompanied by:

- a strong desire to improve
- a capacity to follow through so that knowledge leads, where feasible, to action.

Readers may want to add many other qualities, but this is an attempt to separate the particular values that are necessary for the practice of evidence-based management, not a list of the leadership qualities for managing change.

Avoiding a blame culture

Organisational culture is central to every stage of the learning process – from ensuring that incidents are identified and reported through to embedding the necessary changes deeply into practice. There is evidence that 'safety cultures', where open reporting and balanced analysis are encouraged in principle and by example, can have a positive and quantifiable impact on the performance of organisations. 'Blame cultures' on the other hand can encourage people to cover up errors for fear of retribution and act against the identification of the true causes of failure, because they focus heavily on individual actions and largely ignore the role of underlying systems. The culture of the NHS still errs too much towards the latter.[6]

The report stresses the need to recognise that most adverse events come from system failures and can rarely be attributed just to the mistake of one individual. If the culture is, as the report describes the NHS being, too much of a blame culture, there will not be sufficient effort to try to understand and prevent the system weaknesses that make individual errors more likely.

A good example of what the report is advocating comes from British Airways, who have developed a monitoring system which can identify any departure from normal practice. Such monitoring can be a protection against an accident and be better than waiting until there is a serious accident before trying to identify the cause. Learning from mistakes and malfunctions is of particular importance in organisations where safety is essential, such as airlines and hospitals. One way of assisting such learning is to make it easy for untoward incidents, which could be a sign of a larger safety threat, to be shared without fear of reprisals. British Airways is an example of this and of a particularly rigorous method of safety monitoring: one that is likely to be reassuring to passengers who read this.

Box 7.1: Learning from untoward incidents in British Airways

This case is included for four reasons.

- It is an example of very detailed ongoing monitoring of operations in order to improve safety.
- A way has been found to get this close monitoring of any departures from pre-determined norms accepted by the union.
- Both airlines and health services operate services where safety is of great importance so that effective monitoring systems are highly desirable.
- Lessons from the BA system have been taken into account in establishing the National Patient Safety Agency.

British Airways has developed an unusually good system for safety monitoring, which is accepted by the pilots' union. SESMA (Special Event Search and Master Analysis) is a fully automatic continuous recording of up to 1000 parameters of each and every flight. Instances of flight away from pre-determined 'norms' are automatically detected by the ground replay computer and are called 'events'. Each event is examined by management and statistical trends are noted. If comment is required from the pilot, then he remains anonymous to management, but questions are put to him using the union as a conduit to ensure anonymity. Whatever the pilot says is reported back verbatim.

About 10% of airlines have some form of flight data monitoring, including Cathay, Air France, Lufthansa and Qantas. Research by Skandia (insurance) shows airlines with an established monitoring system have lower accident rates than those who do not.

In a plane, all have a common interest in their mutual safety and hence in a system that helps to provide that. This common interest extends to seeking to prevent behavioural problems. So in most airlines throughout the world there is crew (or cockpit) resource management (CRM), which is a big educational programme about behaviour that upsets other people. This is given on entry and followed up with annual refreshers.

Changing the culture

By now you should know whether the culture of your organisation, and the part of it that you manage, is favourable to the practice of evidence-based management. If you still have doubts, try listing all the words that describe your present culture and compare them with the words that would describe an evidence-based culture. It may be useful to do the same thing for different parts of the organisation to see whether there is a dominant organisational culture or distinct cultures within some common cultural aspects.

The first aim should be to encourage a recognition of the need for improvement and a desire to do so. There may be external factors that provide a spur, such as a scandal or a disaster that focuses attention on how to prevent a similar one. In the private sector, increased competition is often a stimulus to improvement; in the public sector, it will mainly be changes in government policy.

Example carries more conviction than exhortation: 'walk the talk'. So managers who want to change the culture have to illustrate what they mean by the way they act. In earlier chapters, a variety of suggestions for how to do this are given in the 'How to improve' sections. In public organisations where there are lots of meetings, the chair of a meeting has a good opportunity to encourage diversity of opinions and to ensure that critical views are heard. The chair can also ask questions of elucidation to encourage an examination of the nature of the information being put forward.

Recognising that there are useful roles to be played in promoting evidence-based management, and creating such roles, can be another way of trying to change the culture. These are roles that the individual plays in addition to his or her job. They are likely to be ones that he or she may try to play already, but would now have the encouragement and support for doing so. One such role is that of 'gatekeeper'; someone who is a good source of information about what is happening elsewhere and about what has usefully been written on the subject – although it may need different people for the two tasks since they may attract different personalities. The growth of the Internet has made it much easier to search out information. Yet some people will still be more interested in doing so than others and their interest can and should be used.

Another useful role is what Belbin, in his analysis of team roles, called 'monitor evaluator'.[7] He described team roles as: 'a tendency to behave, contribute and interrelate with others at work in distinctive ways'.[8] He describes the monitor evaluator as: 'Sober, strategic and discerning. Sees all options. Judges accurately'. Clearly a person with a useful contribution to make to evidence-based management! But the weaknesses which Belbin describes as an aspect of people who play this role are: lack of drive, an inability to inspire others and a tendency to be overly critical. Explicit in Belbin's theory of team roles is that a good team will consist of people who play different roles that complement each other, so other roles will be necessary to develop a culture of evidence-based management. There need to be people with the relevant knowledge or who, like the gatekeeper, are good at getting it. There needs, too, to be someone with the drive and enthusiasm to persuade others that practising evidence-based management is worth the effort.

Summary

The culture of the organisation, and of powerful groups within it, can make it easier or harder to practise evidence-based management. It is not difficult to assess whether the culture of one's organisation, and of one's own group, is supportive of evidence-based management. Recent reports and lectures have suggested that, by and large, the culture of the NHS is not. So those working in the NHS will need to adopt many of the methods suggested in the 'How to improve' sections at the end of each chapter, including this one. Those who work in other organisations should also review these sections to decide what they may need to improve and how to do it.

How to improve

- Assess the culture of your own organisation, and that of the group with whom you work most closely, using one of the methods suggested.
- Observe what happens in other organisations and ask yourself what that tells you about the culture of your organisation.
- Adopt some of the earlier suggestions for how to improve so as to provide support for a different cultural approach.
- Show by your own actions that you value evidence-based decisions.

References

1 Department of Health (2000) *An Organisation with a Memory*. The Stationery Office, London, p. 72.
2 Southern Birmingham Community Health NHS Trust (2000) *Clinical Governance Annual Report 1999/2000*, p. 11. (This trust was merged with another and became the Birmingham Specialist Community Health NHS Trust.)
3 Shrivastava P (1983) A typology of organizational learning systems. *J Mgmt Studies.* **20**(1): 22.
4 Janis IL (1972) *Victims of Group Think: a psychological study of foreign policy decision and fiascos.* Houghton Mifflin, New York.
5 Leicester G (1999) What works? The role of evidence

in public sector policy and practice (editorial). *Publ Money and Mgmt.* **19**(1): 5.

6 Department of Health (2000) *op. cit.*, p. ix.

7 Belbin M (1993) *Team Roles at Work.* Butterworth-Heinemann, Oxford, p. 23.

8 *ibid.*, p. 25.

8

In conclusion

At the centre of evidence-based management is an obligation and a truism. The managerial obligation is to take the appropriate action arising from the evidence ... The truism is that evidence-based management is not self implementing. It requires considerable effort including, perhaps, change to one's own managerial behaviour.
Peter Homa (1998) *Chief Executive as Management Researcher: the obligation of evidence based management.* Work Paper Series, Henley Management College

Evidence-based management is primarily an attitude of mind that encourages the asking of questions: What? When? Why? Where? How?, and What assumptions are we making? It starts with a belief that improvement is possible and desirable, and that we can learn to do better. This belief should provide the impetus to seeking to reduce the obstacles to practising evidence-based management and to developing the aids to doing so. There are rewards from practising evidence-based management: performance should be better, there should be fewer mistakes and managing should become more interesting too.

Index

AAR *see* after-action reviews
abnormal fluctuations, information
     source 56–7
accountability 10
active/passive learning 126–7
after-action reviews (AAR) 127
agendas, developing own 32
aids, evidence-based management
     22–3
Aintree, University Hospital 99–102
anchor points, information 47–8
appointments systems 65
art, medicine and management as
     11
Asian Cookery Club, learning from
     experience case study 128–32
assumptions 13–14
   questioning 120
   recognising 123–5
   testing 123–5, 140
attention, as resource 34–5
attitude of mind, evidence-based
     management as 5–7, 23, 43, 157

audit, medical records 18, 83–4
Axelsson R 14

Beacon initiatives 146
   decision-making 116
   learning from 63–4
   learning from experience 128–35
   performance monitoring 74–6
   problem tackling 97–102
bed blocking 97–9
Belbin M 153
beliefs about managing 38–9
benchmarking 80–2, 91
benefits, evidence-based
     management 5–6
Berkshire Health Authority 18
   communicating information 51–2
   decision-making case study 24–6
bias, information 48–50
Birmingham Specialist Community
     Health NHS Trust 17–18, 76
   clinical records audit 83–4
blame culture, avoiding 150–1

brainstorming 68–9
British Airways, organisational
    culture 150–1
broad view, information 57–61
budgets, and monitoring 86–8
busyness, buzz from 30, 40

Cambridgeshire Health Authority,
    monitoring 85
cancer appointments, case study
    57–61
Carlson, Sune 30
case studies
    Asian cookery club 128-32
    balanced scorecard 79-80
    bed blocking 97-9
    cancer appointments 57–61
    clinical records audit 83–4
    competency schemes 132–4
    decision-making 24–6
    learning from adverse incidents
        128–32
    physiotherapists 99-102
    primary care 75-6
    problem-tackling 97–9
    training programme 53-4
changes 10–11, 19
    organisational culture 152–3
    organisation's 5, 10, 19
CHI see Commission for Health
    Improvement
choices 35–8, 40–1
Cochrane Centre 8
collaboration 97–9
Collaborative Pathways Project
    Team 97
Commission for Health
    Improvement (CHI) 46
communicating information 51–2
competency schemes, case study
    132–4
complacency 22

complaints, monitoring 85–6
confidentiality, information 81
constraints 35–8
contacts, managers' 52–4, 145–6
context influences 19, 19–23
continuous professional
    development (CPD) 138–9
controversy, EBM 8–10
Cookery Club, learning from
    experience case study 128–32
Cookham Medical Centre,
    performance monitoring 74–6
core idea, evidence-based
    management 15
corroborative evidence 16
CPD see continuous professional
    development
critical incidents, recording 141
Cuban missile crisis, assumptions
    and 123–5
culture
    blame 149
    changing the 152–3
    cynicism 147–8
    NHS 143–4, 149
    organisational 22, 144–55
    research 22
'current best evidence' 14
cynicism culture 147–8

data
    accurate 57–61
    information raw material 43–4,
        57–61
    selecting 49
Davies H 64
decision-making 22
    avoiding 106
    case study 24–6
    defensive avoidance 106
    errors in 95–6
    evaluation 115

group 112–13, 122–3
implementation 117
improve, how to 115–17
improving 93–118, 120, 125
intuition 107–9, 117, 120
leadership and 113–14, 115
lessons from studies 102–6
non-decisions 111–12
outcomes 113–14, 125
politics in 110–11
stages 94–6
tactics 102–6, 115
timescale 13
uncertainty 113
decision types 13
defensive avoidance, decision-
    making 106
delay, knowledge adoption 63–5
Delphi technique, decision-making
    69
demands, managerial 35–8
devil's advocate technique,
    decision-making 69, 117
differences, evidence-based
    management/EBM 12–13

education, influence of 20
Einstein A 68
empirical evidence 120–1
Enthoven, Alain 77–8
evaluation
    and decision-making 115
    prioritisation process 25–6
    project 131–2
evidence
    availability 11
    corroborative 16
    defined 13–14
    empirical 120–1
    in management 13–15
    meaning of 8–10
    nature of 12

reliability of 15–17, 120–1
evidence-based management
    as attitude of mind 5–7, 23, 43,
        157
    benefits 5–6
    cf. EBM 10–13
    core idea 15
    defined 6
    influences 18–23
    learning to practise 119–42
    meaning of 14
    obligation 157
    obstacles 20–3
    overview 5–27
    roles 152–3
    truism 157
    values underlying 149
Evidence-based Medicine 8
evidence-based medicine (EBM) 7–
    13
    controversy 8–10
    defined 6, 23
    lessons from 7–10
    as link to evidence-based
        management 17–18
experience
    information source 55
    learning from 126–37
    value attached to 13

failings, overcoming management
    5, 7
fashions, management 31–2, 40
feedback 54, 121–3, 127–8, 141
fluctuations, information source 56–
    7
fragmented managerial work 30
Frimley Park Hospital, cancer
    appointments case study 57–61

GANNT charts, event scheduling
    tool 98

general practice 74-6
  information sharing 146
Good Hospital Guide 78
GP *see* general practice
Greenwich Healthcare NHS Trust,
    problem-tackling case study
    97–9
group decision-making 112–13
  learning in 122–3
'group think' concept 146–7

hospitals
  Good Hospital Guide 78
  Nottingham City Hospital NHS
    Trust 132–4
  Tampere University Hospital 79–
    80
  University Hospital Aintree 99–
    102

ideas, generating, decision-making
    tactic 103
imagination, and knowledge 67–9
*Imaginisation: the art of creative
    management* 68
implementation
  decision-making 117
  knowledge 62
  tactics 104–5
improve, how to
  decision-making 115–17
  learning to practise evidence-
    based management 140–1
  monitoring performance 90–1
  organisational culture 154
  using information and
    knowledge 70
In Search of Excellence 55
In Search of Management 39
inertia
  information 45, 47
  using knowledge 65, 134

inferences 49–50
influences, evidence-based
    management 18–23
information
  anchor points 47–8
  availability 46
  bias 48–50
  broad view 57–61
  communicating 51–2
  confidentiality 81
  forms 48
  importance 5
  improve, how to 70
  inaccurate 16–17
  inertia 45, 47
  management 22
  misinformation 46
  obstacles 45–7
  obtaining 45–7
  organising 56–7
  overwhelming 45, 47
  probabilities 48
  quality 45–7
  quality-related 77
  as raw material 43–4
  research 52
  selection and use 48–50
  social aspect, information sharing
    52–4, 136–7, 145–6
  sources 50–61, 120, 136–7, 145–6
  trends 49, 56–7
  using 43–71
intervention, decision-making tactic
    103, 104–5
intuition 20
  dangers 109
  decision-making 107–9, 117, 120
  experience 107–8
  knowledge 120
  management 20
  nurturing 108
  purposes 107–8

Irvine, Sir Donald 144

Janis IL 106
job influences, evidence-based
    management 19–23
job, managing the 29–41
job model 35–8
Journal of Nursing Management 14–
    15
judgements, value of 20, 22, 49–50

key events, information source 56
Knowing-Doing Gap 64–5
knowledge
    academic/practical 61–2
    adoption delay 63–5
    appraisal 62
    and imagination 67–9
    implementation 62
    improve, how to 70
    inertia 65, 134
    management 17–18, 61–2, 65–7
    marketing 62
    production 62
    sharing 65–7, 145–6
    storage 62
    using 43–71
Knowledge Space 136
Kotter, John 32

leadership
    and decision-making 113–14,
        115
    team leader training 53–4
learning
    active/passive 126–7
    from experience 126–37
    lifelong learning 138–9
    from the past 135–7
    to practise evidence-based
        management 119–42
    from research 137–8

social aspect 52–4, 136–7, 145–6
    sources 126–38
    topics 119–21
Leicester, Graham 147–8
lifelong learning 138–9
limitations in reasoning 47–50
London Ambulance Service 53-4

management
    evidence in 13–15
    failings, overcoming 5, 7
    fashions 31–2, 40
    fragmented work 30
    seductions of 30–3
Management Challenges for the 21st
    Century 56–7
managerial job model 35–8
managing, beliefs about 38–9
managing the job 29–41
Mann L 106
mental maps 120, 123
methods available, evidence-based
    practice 12–13
misinformation 46
monitoring 120
    British Airways system 150–1
    budgets and 86–8
    complaints 85–6
    organisational monitoring
        systems 50, 73–92
    performance 18, 73–92
    reliability of 86–8
Morgan, Gareth 68
Myers Briggs test 109

National Patient Safety Agency
    151
Nelson LS 82
NHS culture 143–4, 149
non-decisions, decision-making
    111–12
Noordegraaf M 35

Nottingham City Hospital NHS
    Trust
  competency schemes case study
      132–4
  learning from experience
      example 132–4
Nutley S 64
Nutt, Paul 102–6

objective setting, decision-making
    tactic 103, 115
objectives 93
obstacles
  evidence-based management 20–
      3
  information 45–7
opportunities, vs. threats 47–8
organisation, values of the 55–6
Organisation with a Memory 89–90,
    126–7
organisational context, evidence-
    based management 19, 19–23
organisational culture 22, 144–55
  improve, how to 154
organisational monitoring systems
    50, 73–92
organising time 33–4
Osler, William 63
outcomes, decision-making 113–14,
    125
outpatients 87
overview, evidence-based
    management 5–27

participation, decision-making
    tactic 104–5
Patient Administration System
    (PAS) 59–61
people, as information source 52–4,
    136–7, 145–6
performance, improving 120
performance monitoring 18, 73–92
  improve, how to 90–1

personal factor influences,
    evidence-based management
    19–23
persuasion, decision-making tactic
    105
play areas 31, 40
politics, in decision-making 110–11
primary care *see* general practice
prioritisation process, evaluation
    25–6
prioritising 34–5, 93
problem solving, decision-making
    tactic 103
problems
  identifying 116
  nature of 12
  recognising 95, 96
  tackling 97–102
project, evaluation 131–2
psychology 16, 22

questioning approach 7
questionnaires 122

randomised controlled trials (RCTs)
    15–16
rationale, evidence-based practice
    12
RCTs *see* randomised controlled
    trials
reasoning, human limitations in 47–
    50
record keeping 40
  audit of medical 18
  clinical records audit 83–4
  critical incidents 141
referrals
  systems improvement 97–102
  TWR 59–61
  waiting lists 99–102
reflection
  management 20
  reflective practice 121, 126

reliability
  evidence 15–17, 120–1
  monitoring 86–8
research
  applied 21
  culture 22
  information 52
  learning from 137–8
reviews 140, 141
  AAR 127
roles, evidence-based management
    152–3

scorecards, performance
    monitoring 78–80, 91
seductions of management 30–3
shaped, vs. shaping 29–30, 32–3
sharing, knowledge 65–7, 145–6
Shipman, Dr Harold 57, 75–6, 88
similarities, evidence-based
    management/EBM 10–11
social aspect, learning/information
    sharing 52–4, 136–7, 145–6
solution searching, decision-making
    116–17
sources
  information 50–61, 120, 136–7,
    145–6
  learning 126–38
space, making 35–8
strengths 39–40
success, measuring 73–92
suggestion schemes 141
surprises, avoiding bad 88–90

tactics
  decision-making 102–6, 115
  implementation 104–5

Tampere University Hospital 79–80
target setting/monitoring 79–80
team
  leader training 53–4
  roles 153
Thinking in Time 135
threats, vs. opportunities 47–8
threshold concept, information
    source 57
time
  making 33–4
  management 33
  pressures 11, 20–1, 22, 29, 45
  use of 38
timescales, decision-making 13
training, team leader 53–4
trends, information 49, 56–7
troubleshooting pleasures 31, 40
two-week referral (TWR) 59–61

uncertainty, decision-making 113
University Hospital Aintree 99–102

values
  experience, attached to 13
  of judgements 20, 22, 49–50
  of the organisation 55–6
  underlying evidence-based
    management 149

waiting lists 65, 87, 97, 99–102
walking around, management by
    46
Watson, Tony 39
weaknesses 39–40
Web, information source 50–2
written information sources 50–2

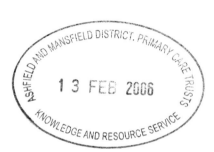

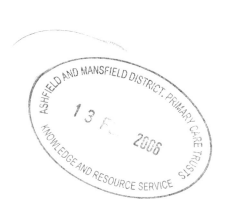

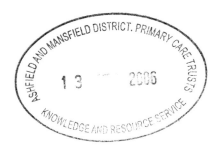